Seasonal
Affective Disorder
FOR
DUMMIES®

Seasonal Affective Disorder

FOR

DUMMIES®

by Laura L. Smith, PhD, and
Charles H. Elliott, PhD

Wiley Publishing, Inc.

Seasonal Affective Disorder For Dummies®

Published by
Wiley Publishing, Inc.
111 River St.
Hoboken, NJ 07030-5774
www.wiley.com

For general information on our other products and services, please contact our Customer Care Department within the U.S. at 800-762-2974, outside the U.S. at 317-572-3993, or fax 317-572-4002.

For technical support, please visit www.wiley.com/techsupport.

Wiley also publishes its books in a variety of electronic formats. Some content that appears in print may not be available in electronic books.

Library of Congress Control Number: 2007935016

ISBN: 978-0-470-13999-8

Manufactured in the United States of America

10 9 8 7 6 5 4 3 2 1

WILEY

About the Authors

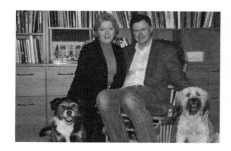

Laura L. Smith, PhD is a clinical psychologist in private practice in Corrales, New Mexico. She provides consultation to attorneys, school districts, and governmental agencies. She specializes in the assessment and treatment of both adults and children with depression, anxiety, and other emotional disorders. In addition, she's presented on cognitive therapy and mental health issues to both national and international audiences.

Dr. Smith is coauthor of *Anxiety and Depression Workbook For Dummies* (Wiley), *Depression For Dummies* (Wiley), *Overcoming Anxiety For Dummies* (Wiley), *Hollow Kids: Recapturing the Soul of a Generation Lost to the Self-Esteem Myth* (Prima), and *Why Can't I Be the Parent I Want to Be?* (New Harbinger Publications).

Charles H. Elliott, PhD is a clinical psychologist and a member of the faculty at Fielding Graduate University. He's a Founding Fellow in the Academy of Cognitive Therapy, an internationally recognized organization that certifies cognitive therapists. He has a part time private practice in Corrales, New Mexico, that specializes in the treatment of anxiety and depression. In addition, he's written many articles and book chapters in the area of cognitive behavior therapies. He's made numerous presentations nationally and internationally on new developments in assessment and therapy of emotional disorders. He's coauthor of *Anxiety and Depression Workbook For Dummies* (Wiley), *Depression For Dummies* (Wiley), *Overcoming Anxiety For Dummies* (Wiley), *Why Can't I Get What I Want?* (Davies-Black), *Why Can't I Be the Parent I Want to Be?* (New Harbinger Publications), and *Hollow Kids* (Prima).

Drs. Smith and Elliott are available for speaking engagements and workshops. You can visit their Web site at www.PsychAuthors.com.

Dedication

To all our families and especially to Lauren, Alaina, and Carter.

Authors' Acknowledgments

We want to thank our excellent editors at Wiley: Stephen R. Clark, Mike Baker, and Carrie Burchfield, as well as our agents Elizabeth and Ed Knappman.

A special thanks to all the fine folks in Homer, Alaska, for their insights and thoughts about SAD. This thanks includes the people at NAMI, psychologist, Dr. John Gamache, and all the unsuspecting citizens we interviewed.

We also want to acknowledge Ricardo Castillo Ayuso, Lorena Gamboa Ancona, and their wonderful students at the University Universidad Autónoma de Yucatán for inspiration and enthusiasm.

We appreciate the hard work of Erika Hansen, future novelist and bibliographer extraordinaire. Thanks to Scott Love of Softek, LLC, for his usual care and expertise in keeping our computers running. Similarly, we thank Howard Eckstein of MCD Electronics, Inc. for explaining the technical aspects of light. And Trevor Wolfe for his unflagging support as well as his translation skills.

To Doctors Brad Richards and Jeanne Czajka from the Cognitive Behavioral Institute of Albuquerque, thanks for listening. We appreciate Dr. Brenda Wolfe for her encouragement and collaboration on future endeavors. Finally, we thank Frank Gonzales of the Center for Body-Mind Awareness for keeping our bodies flexible and our minds focused.

Publisher's Acknowledgments

We're proud of this book; please send us your comments through our Dummies online registration form located at www.dummies.com/register/.

Some of the people who helped bring this book to market include the following:

Acquisitions, Editorial, and Media Development

Project Editor: Stephen R. Clark

Acquisitions Editor: Mike Baker

Copy Editor: Carrie A. Burchfield

Technical Editor:
Rebecca Moredock Mueller, MD

Editorial Manager: Christine Meloy Beck

Editorial Assistants: Erin Calligan Mooney, Joe Niesen, Leeann Haney, and David Lutton

Cover Photos: © ImageState/Alamy

Cartoons: Rich Tennant
(www.the5thwave.com)

Composition Services

Project Coordinator: Adrienne Martinez

Layout and Graphics: Carl Byers, Joyce Haughey, Laura Pence, Alicia B. South

Anniversary Logo Design: Richard Pacifico

Proofreaders: Susan Moritz, Toni Settle

Indexer: Potomac Indexing, LLC

Publishing and Editorial for Consumer Dummies

    Diane Graves Steele, Vice President and Publisher, Consumer Dummies

    Joyce Pepple, Acquisitions Director, Consumer Dummies

    Kristin A. Cocks, Product Development Director, Consumer Dummies

    Michael Spring, Vice President and Publisher, Travel

    Kelly Regan, Editorial Director, Travel

Publishing for Technology Dummies

    Andy Cummings, Vice President and Publisher, Dummies Technology/General User

Composition Services

    Gerry Fahey, Vice President of Production Services

    Debbie Stailey, Director of Composition Services

Contents at a Glance

Table of Contents

Introduction

Seasonal affective disorder (SAD) is a type of depression that comes and goes as seasons change. The most prevalent form of SAD arrives in the fall and winter and lifts during the spring and summer. Many experts believe that reduced sunlight during the winter months triggers SAD. Interestingly, the number of SAD cases increases in populations farther from the equator where winter nights are especially long.

We like to travel. We also like to write. Combining the two is even better. When we considered the request to write *Seasonal Affective Disorder For Dummies,* we immediately thought about the travel implications. Obviously, we needed to trek to higher latitudes to research the topic and talk with people who actually suffer from SAD. A fall trip north to Alaska appeared essential. Mush!

Geography isn't our forte; after all, we're psychologists. Looking at the map, Alaska seemed to be just a bit North of Seattle. The plane ride from Dallas took a surprisingly long six and a half hours. (Okay, so Alaska is farther North of Seattle than we thought.) We prepared for the cold by purchasing insulated shoes, coats, gloves — the works! We needed none of this cold weather attire in New Mexico, but we were prepared for blizzard conditions.

Apparently, in our haste, we forgot to research Alaskan climate well enough. In Homer, Alaska, during this particular September, the weather was shockingly wonderful! The sun shined brightly, and the temperature hovered in the low 60s. It wasn't exactly tropical, but our winter attire remained in our suitcases. Nonetheless, we were having an enlightening time talking to the locals about their real-world experiences with SAD. And the views of the ocean, mountains, and glaciers rival anything we've ever seen. How could anyone get depressed in a beautiful and glorious place such as Homer, Alaska? More on that later.

Our fall Alaskan trip was followed by a tropical winter trip to Yucatan, Mexico. (Hmm, isn't "tropical winter" an oxymoron?) But we clearly needed to venture south, close to the equator, for contrast purposes. Darn, another grueling research trip. And indeed Yucatan was quite a contrast to Alaska. The people of Yucatan are as warm and friendly as the weather. And they rarely suffer from SAD.

In this book, we provide you with our collective wisdom about SAD. Our knowledge comes from clinical experience, field and other research, and the composite stories of people battling SAD.

About This Book

This book is about SAD. Our goals are to help you understand this problem, give you strategies for feeling better, and, in some cases, tell you what you can do for someone you care about who has SAD. Our intention is to share the latest and most accurate information about SAD, as well as provide tools for effectively dealing with SAD.

At the same time we want to make you smile. You find dashes of humor interjected from time to time throughout the writing. We want to brighten your day with a little light fun while also fully respecting the seriousness of struggling with SAD.

You very well may be reading this book as a source of help for your own battle with SAD. Please feel free to write in the book as you read, unless of course you checked it out from the library; in that case, please don't write in the book. In either case, you may want to take notes in a notebook. Use the notebook to complete the exercises in the chapters and write out your feelings, thoughts, and reactions to them as you go.

Conventions Used in This Book

The following conventions are used throughout the book to make things consistent and easy to understand:

- **Boldface text: Bold** text is used to highlight the important concepts of bulleted lists (like this list you're reading right now) and the action steps of numbered lists.

- **Italics:** New terms appear in *italics* and are closely followed by an easy-to-understand definition.

- **Jargon:** Occasionally we use *jargon*. If you hang around psychologists or psychiatrists very long you know that they tend to use a lot of technical terms and phrases — jargon — such as PTSD, diagnostic criteria, DSM, medical model, contingencies, schemas, MDD, and so on. Shrinks aren't smarter than other people, they just use a different vocabulary.

  We promise to try and use as little jargon as possible. The primary technical term we use is SAD, which is merely an acronym for seasonal affective disorder. We carefully define SAD in Chapters 1 and 2. A few other professional terms and acronyms pop up, but we really do keep it to a minimum (we hope). Don't worry; each term is defined as you read, so you aren't left in the dark.

- ✔ **Stories:** Throughout the book, you read about individuals who experience symptoms of SAD and related disorders. You can be assured that these stories accurately illustrate the feelings, thoughts, and actions of real people. However, the individual examples are composites drawn from people and clients we've known, yet the people are thoroughly disguised to protect their privacy. Any resemblance to any person, whether alive or deceased, is entirely coincidental. We **bold** the names of people the first time they appear in order to alert you to the fact that we are presenting an example.

- ✔ **Web addresses:** All Web addresses appear in `monofont`. Please note that at times a Web address may be long and may break over two lines. If this breakage occurs, make sure to type the address in your Web browser exactly as it appears in the book without including extra spaces at the end of a line.

What You're Not to Read

Well, of course we wouldn't spend this much time writing this darn book if we didn't think it was all important! However, the truth is, you really don't have to read all of it. For example, if you don't care that much about what may cause SAD, you don't have to read the material on that topic. Furthermore, sidebars (the gray shaded boxes) and text marked by the icon "Technical Stuff" throughout the book offer interesting or technical tidbits that may or may not interest you. We think they're pretty cool, but then again, we're shrinks.

Foolish Assumptions

This idea may seem foolish, but we presume that if you're reading this paragraph, you've picked up the book and are trying to decide whether to read or buy it. If that's the case, you probably have some interest in SAD.

Here are some other assumptions that we've made about you:

- ✔ Maybe you struggle with SAD or are close to someone who does.
- ✔ You want to do something about feeling better, especially during the winter months.
- ✔ You're intelligent but don't know a lot about SAD.
- ✔ Winter is probably not your favorite time of year.

If you've gotten this far, we enthusiastically recommend that you buy and read the book (or check it out of the library). We promise to make it as useful and painless as possible. Finally, buy 20 copies for your friends!

How This Book Is Organized

This book is divided into six parts. Each one is distinct and covers important information. Let us tell you a little about each part.

Part 1: Detecting and Dealing with SAD

Chapter 1 describes typical symptoms of SAD. We overview the possible causes of SAD as well as highlights of the major treatment approaches for SAD. Chapter 2 goes into more detail about symptoms and helps you figure out if you or someone close to you has SAD. Next, we talk about who's most likely to come down with a case of SAD and why that happens. Finally, this part concludes by giving you information about when, where, and how to get professional help if you need it.

Part II: Examining the Biological Treatments for SAD

In Chapter 5, you discover the pros and cons of light therapy, the first treatment developed specifically for SAD. While this approach does work for many SAD sufferers, it may not be for you. In the next chapter, we help you decide whether medication is a good choice for you. We tell you about the various medications available as well as describe their possible side effects. Chapter 7 discusses the role of diet in SAD. Often, increased, unhealthy cravings for food, and sometimes drugs or alcohol, form a significant part of the picture with SAD. Finally, Chapter 8 reviews the various alternative treatments for SAD. While some of these alternatives look promising, others we recommend avoiding.

Part III: Shifting SAD Thoughts

In this part, you look into how your thinking affects the way you feel and, conversely, how the way you feel affects the way you think. You may assume that thoughts wouldn't have much to do with SAD, but that's not the case. We show you how SAD can distort your thinking, making the problem worse. We also provide methods for changing flawed SAD thinking into better thinking. We give some strategies for conquering upsetting emotions when they occur in spite of your best attempts to calm distressing thoughts. And you get a variety of ways for managing and reducing the stress of SAD.

Part IV: Changing SAD Behaviors

Part IV helps you take action against SAD by using the tools of behavior therapy. You discover how to get yourself up and moving again, one small step at a time. You also read about sleep — how to get better sleep without sleeping too much or too little. Exercise is also important, and one whole chapter is devoted to showing you good exercises to fend off SAD. And you also need to have some fun! The last chapter in this part allows you to feel good about putting fun back into your life.

Part V: Life after SAD

Chapter 17 reviews a number of ways for fending off SAD relapse. Unfortunately, the relapse rate for all kinds of depression is a little scary. However, being aware and prepared can substantially reduce that risk. Chapter 18 describes mindful acceptance, an ancient approach to recovery that's recently been rediscovered. Finally, in this part, we offer a recipe for finding ongoing fulfillment and happiness even in the face of sadness. You see that happiness is more than a mere absence of SAD.

Part VI: The Part of Tens

The quick hitting chapters in The Part of Tens provide tips and tidbits for bringing more light into your life, pulling out of a bad mood, and helping children or somebody you care about who has SAD. Go to these chapters when you want quick information about these topics.

This part also includes the appendixes. The first appendix gives you some blank forms for some of the exercises described throughout this book. Feel free to copy them for your own use. The second appendix lists a variety of additional resources for understanding and dealing with SAD.

Icons Used in This Book

Throughout this book, you see icons that enhance your reading pleasure and flag special types of info. So, when you meet one of these pictures, consider the following:

This icon appears in order to highlight a specific idea or insight relevant to SAD.

You see this icon to emphasize something of importance such as a skill you need to practice.

Watch out for this icon. It alerts you to information you need to know in order to avoid trouble.

This icon tells you that the following information is a little technical. Thus, it isn't really critical if you don't like knowing all the details.

You see this icon when a questionnaire or checklist appears in a chapter for you to complete or that's shown as an example of a completed form.

Where to Go from Here

This book is comprehensive, but you don't need to read every chapter and every sentence. Furthermore, you can start just about anywhere you want. We organized the material so you can read straight through the book from beginning to end or just look up information you want in the Table of Contents.

We hope that reading this book thoroughly informs you about SAD and provides state-of-the-art tools for dealing with it. However, we suggest that you get professional help if you feel helpless, hopeless, or suicidal. Also, if you feel stuck despite your best efforts, it's most likely time to turn to someone else for help.

If you do choose to work with a mental health professional, this book is still a useful adjunct to the work you do with that person. Finally, be sure to check with your family doctor for a complete physical — sometimes depression is due to a purely physical problem.

Part I
Detecting and Dealing with SAD

The 5th Wave   By Rich Tennant

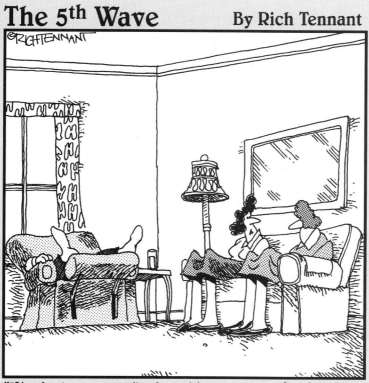

"His doctor prescribed antidepressants for his SAD, but Dave prefers his own recline-a-therapy."

In this part . . .

You get an overview of the symptoms and signs of seasonal affective disorders (SAD). We cover the treatment options and tell you about the other emotional problems that may look like SAD but aren't. We also provide information about who gets SAD and why. This part concludes with advice about determining whether you need professional help for SAD and how to find a mental health professional if you do need assistance.

Chapter 1

Opening Up the Curtains on SAD

*P*eople with seasonal affective disorder (SAD) dread the turn from fall to winter. Darkness on the outside brings depression on the inside. People with SAD don't look forward to cozy nights in front of a roaring fire, skiing, making snowmen, or celebrating holidays. Instead, they simply hope and pray that they can muddle through until spring.

Most scientists believe that the primary cause of SAD is diminished sunlight that accompanies the shorter days in the winter. For many people, reduced light triggers changes that reverberate throughout their bodies and minds, causing their moods to darken (see Chapter 3 for a review of other causes of SAD).

In this chapter, we open the curtains on SAD, illuminating both the symptoms and treatments for SAD. With this insight in hand, you'll know if you suffer from SAD and how to overcome the misery if you have it.

Getting to Know SAD

There's more to SAD than changing seasons. SAD is a real form of depression that can seriously impact a sufferer. Moods associated with SAD can be so dark that the person starts missing work, withdraws from people, and in rare cases, contemplates suicide.

SAD is more serious than bad moods related to cold weather or cloudy days. People with SAD usually report overwhelming feelings of fatigue, seriously depressed moods, cravings for carbohydrates, and disturbed sleep. These symptoms tend to endure through the winter months and improve in the spring.

How do you know if you have SAD? For starters, how do you feel about the seasons? Are you a summer or a winter person? We have a quiz for you.

Check off which of the following items apply to you:

❏ I like summer more than winter.

❏ I'm more active in the summer.

❏ I don't like the shorter days of winter as much as longer days in the summer.

❏ I don't like leaving work at 5:00 p.m. when it's already getting dark.

❏ I really enjoy the feeling of the first warm days of spring.

❏ I spend more time outside in the summer.

❏ I tend to gain a couple of pounds in the winter.

Did you answer yes to many if not all of the items? Guess what? If you did, that's pretty darn normal. *Most* people express a little preference for the summer and its longer days. And *most* people are a little more active in the summer than the winter.

The point we're trying to make is that a mere preference for the summer versus the winter doesn't mean you have SAD. In fact, your favorite season may be fall with its cooling temperatures and colorful foliage, yet you suffer from SAD that hits you hard after the last leaf falls. SAD is a condition in which the sufferers experience a major deterioration in moods that seems to come and go with the seasons (winter is especially problematic for the vast majority of SAD sufferers). Typical symptoms include

✔ Deep sadness

✔ Fatigue, excessive sleep

✔ Feelings of regret

✔ Loss of energy

✔ Loss of motivation

✔ Sense of worthlessness

✔ Weight gain (more than just a couple of pounds)

✔ Withdrawal from people

If these signs sound like what you're experiencing, you may have SAD. Read Chapter 2 for more specific information about SAD symptoms and how they're similar to and different from other emotional problems.

While the symptoms of SAD are more intense during the colder, darker months, they can have an impact at other times of the year. A few people have a form of SAD that's more intense in the brighter, sunnier months. As with any mood disorder or emotional problem, the causes can be complex requiring varied approaches for relief and cure. If you suffer from SAD and have tried one or two therapies without positive results, don't give up! There's more than one way to bring the light back into your life. We share them with you throughout this book.

Finding Out What to Do about SAD

We have good news for you. If you or someone you know has SAD, much can be done to alleviate the suffering. In fact, many good options for treating this condition exist today. At the same time, many of these options have been around a surprisingly long time (see the nearby sidebar "Ancient wisdom").

In this book, we bring you information on the range of treatments that are likely to be helpful for SAD. These options include cognitive-behavior therapy that focuses on how to change both your thoughts and behavior in healthy ways. We also look at the biological factors behind SAD that affect your moods. Biologically focused treatments include light therapy, medication, diet, hormones, and supplements.

Using your mind to overcome SAD

A highly effective way of alleviating SAD involves using the mind to re-establish good moods, increase energy, and instill hope. Again, the mind, body, and environment interact. When depressed people figure out how to think in non-depressed ways, their brains show improvements in functioning. See the sidebar "Changing thinking changes brains."

In the 1950s, Dr. Aaron T. Beck developed the first therapy designed to help people with depression change how they think. Literally hundreds of studies since that time have shown that this therapy works very well for depression and a host of other emotional problems. Interestingly, no one applied this approach to the treatment of SAD for almost another 50 years. That neglect may have been due to the fact that most folks figured that because a lack of light was the major assumed cause of SAD, light would provide the major avenue to the alleviation of the problem.

Ancient wisdom

Psychologist Steve Ilardi at the University of Kansas wondered why so many people suffer from depression. Almost a fourth of all Americans suffer from a type of depression at some point in their lives (including SAD, which most professionals consider to be a type of depression). Dr. Ilardi thought that the changes brought about by modern living may be responsible for the increase in dark moods. The fact that depression is more common in developed countries and in urban settings provided a clue.

He and his research team looked at factors that have changed over the centuries that may explain why so many people suffer. These factors include the following:

✔ People in ancient cultures, for the most part, got more exercise.

✔ They also got more exposure to light.

✔ They woke up when the sun came up and went to sleep when darkness fell.

✔ They lived in groups and didn't have a lot of time for whining, brooding, and complaining.

✔ Survival took up most of their time and attention; after all, it's not easy fighting off saber toothed tigers.

The Therapeutic Lifestyle Change program was developed based on these observations. The program encourages people with depression to get more exercise, light, and *omega-3 fatty acids* (an essential fatty acid that's been depleted from many modern diets). People in the program are also encouraged to become more socially connected and stop thinking about how bad things are for them. The treatment, although still in the very early stages of research, has been unusually successful in reducing depressive symptoms. Interestingly, *all* these suggestions (and more) can be found throughout this book.

All emotional disorders, including SAD, have multiple causes (see Chapter 3 for more about the causes of SAD), and they can be treated in various ways. So, finally research established that cognitive therapy worked well for the alleviation of SAD. Furthermore, willingness to stick with cognitive therapy may be greater than for light therapy, and cognitive therapy may do more to prevent relapse than lights.

See Chapters 9 and 10 for more information about how you can use cognitive therapy if you have SAD. And see the sidebar "When thoughts lead to SAD" for recent findings about how attitudes can make you vulnerable to SAD.

Tinkering with a SAD body

Emotional problems don't exist just in your mind; they impact your body simultaneously. And vice versa! Your moods actually come about from an interaction of your thoughts, the environment, and your physiology. So, while changing your thinking about SAD is a significant component to getting better, physical changes can also help. One of the major approaches for treating SAD involves therapies specifically aimed at influencing biological processes. The biological strategies include the following:

✔ **Alternatives:** The hormone melatonin is an especially promising possibility for re-regulating the biological clock that gets out of synch with SAD. Omega-3 oils, found in fish, seem to help in the treatment of SAD and other types of depression as well. However, some natural alternatives provide more hype than hope. See Chapter 8 for a full discussion of alternative biological approaches to the treatment of SAD.

✔ **Diet:** Changes in diet aren't usually considered a front-line treatment for SAD. However, people with SAD complain about carbohydrate cravings, weight gain, and energy loss. Changes in diet may help with all these problems. See Chapter 7 for more information about how to consider diet in your game plan for addressing SAD.

✔ **Light therapy:** This treatment was the first designed to target SAD specifically. Light therapy involves exposure to intensely bright lights for a period of 30 or more minutes each day. Most people with SAD can expect improvement with light therapy within a couple of weeks, sometimes even sooner. See Chapter 5 for the ins and outs of light therapy.

✔ **Medications:** Anti-depressant medications have helped millions of people overcome depression. They appear to be quite helpful in the treatment of SAD, too, although the research on their effectiveness is somewhat more limited for this application.

One medication, Wellbutrin, is the first to have received specific FDA approval for the treatment of SAD. Wellbutrin may target SAD symptoms more directly than other medications, and it's been used to prevent future recurrences of the disorder. Furthermore, Wellbutrin usually decreases appetite, thereby alleviating the weight gain that many people with SAD experience. See Chapter 6 for more information about medications for the treatment of SAD.

Changing thinking changes brains

Depressed people have negative thoughts about themselves, the world, and the future. After successful treatment with antidepressant medication, depressive thinking usually subsides. Brains of depressed people look different before treatment and after treatment with anti-depressant medication.

Cognitive therapy, which involves changing the way people think, has also been found to be highly effective in the treatment of depression.

A group of researchers wondered if the brains of people treated with cognitive therapy changed like the brains of people who'd been treated only with medication. So, researchers scanned the brains of a group of people before and after 15 to 20 sessions of cognitive therapy. For those people in the group that benefited from cognitive therapy, pre- and post-brain scans showed significant differences. Like anti-depressant medication, cognitive therapy changes thinking and *also* changes the brain.

Making moves against SAD

SAD makes you feel tired, unenthusiastic, and unmotivated. Those feelings lead to procrastination and isolation. Not getting things done leads to guilt and being alone leads to loneliness. Both increase SAD. It's a vicious cycle, and that's not good.

So, one way to treat SAD is with an increase in activity — and we mean a lot of activity — the more the better. Activities for alleviating SAD fall under two major categories:

✔ **Mastery:** These activities give you a sense of accomplishment. They're usually a little challenging. However, when you have SAD, you need to give yourself a little extra credit even for small tasks, such as washing the dishes, balancing your checkbook, or cleaning out a closet because even those tasks are more challenging than they would be without SAD in your life.

✔ **Pleasure:** These activities are for the sole purpose of experiencing enjoyment. Unfortunately, if you have a case of SAD, nothing looks like it can give you pleasure. But if you make yourself do a variety of these activities anyway, you're likely to find enjoyment seeping slowly back into your life. So consider going to a movie, taking a walk, or visiting friends.

We recommend that you take on a variety of activities from both the mastery and pleasure categories. And if you find things to do outside, that's even better because you get more exposure to light — sort of a double bonus play.

Whether you choose activities that give you a sense of accomplishment, pleasure, or both, we recommend that you start small. Don't take on things that feel outside of your reach. Just be consistent with your effort to participate and you'll get there.

Exercise is a special type of activity that can give you a sense of mastery, but quite possibly pleasure as well. The pleasure part usually comes after you've been engaging in exercise a while. Exercise releases endorphins — natural body chemicals that feel good. Exercise seems to work about as well for depression or SAD as medications, light, and thought therapy. When it comes to exercise, you have a lot of possibilities to choose from. See Chapter 15 for information about your exercise options as well as how to get yourself motivated to do it.

Knowing when to get help

Self-help has been shown to work very well for depression, SAD, and many other emotional problems. You may find that reading this book and working on what we suggest (such as light therapy, increased activities, and thinking differently) snaps you right back to feeling good again. But sometimes people need a little extra help.

The decision to seek help depends on a variety of issues. Making that decision certainly isn't a sign of weakness or laziness. It's a tough but brave decision to make.

Please seek professional help *immediately* if you have any of the following symptoms:

- ✔ Feeling as if there's nothing you can do to better your situation
- ✔ Feeling totally hopeless
- ✔ Feeling unable to perform your usual responsibilities
- ✔ Feelings of desperation
- ✔ Hearing voices
- ✔ Seeing things that aren't really there
- ✔ Serious weight loss
- ✔ Thoughts of ending your life
- ✔ Very weird, unusual thoughts

Even if you don't have serious symptoms like the ones above, you may simply prefer to get a little help. Just as you may hire a tutor for Spanish or a personal trainer for sticking with an exercise regimen, you may want a therapist to help guide you through the process of getting better. The different kinds of nonprofessional and professional help are covered in Chapter 4.

Going from SAD to Glad

Our primary purpose in writing this book is to help you erase SAD from your life. And we give you ways of accomplishing that goal as well as prevent the reoccurrence of SAD in the future. But we can't resist trying to take you a little further.

If you get past your SAD, that's wonderful. Some people recover from SAD or other types of depression and feel great. But others are left feeling a little flat — not bad, not sad, but a little empty. It's like SAD consumed their spirit and energy. Winning the battle of SAD leaves them feeling a lack of purpose and meaning.

If this state of affairs applies to you, we have some thoughts to share. You won't find solid, lasting happiness by seeking momentary pleasures, money, or the fountain of youth. On the other hand, you can discover sustainable peace and satisfaction from your life.

The path for getting there includes what we call the "Five F's":

- **Feeling grateful:** If you're reading this book, that means you can read! Appreciate what you take for granted, like reading. Someone cared enough to send you to school and teach you to read. Your life no doubt has many other gifts that are all too easy to overlook. We recommend that you notice these endowments and allow yourself to savor them.

- **Finding forgiveness:** Anger and revenge aren't good for your health or your spirit. When you forgive others who've wronged you, you give yourself the gift of peace and serenity.

- **Focusing on the present:** People make themselves miserable when they focus on anxieties and worries about the future as well as regrets and guilt from the past. Few present moments are all that bad so figure out how to focus on now.

- **Forging meaning through good works:** People report feeling that their lives are more meaningful when they donate to worthy causes, pitch in to help others, and contribute to the betterment of the planet. Make a decision to volunteer something of yourself to others. You'll be glad you did.

- **Forming better connections:** Humans are social creatures. Research says that people with good social supports and relationships get sick less often and feel better emotionally.

See Chapters 18 and 19 for more information about all the above points.

Chapter 2

Is It SAD or Something Else?

In This Chapter

▶ Detecting degrees of depression and mood disorders

▶ Figuring out when depression is SAD

▶ Dealing with thoughts of suicide

*W*hen the warmth of summer fades and the days grow short and cold, are you dogged by seasonal affective disorder (SAD) or something else? It would be nice if you could diagnose SAD and other forms of depression by pricking your finger, placing a drop of blood on a piece of paper, and getting a reading from a portable device like a glucose monitor. However, it's not that easy. SAD or any type of depression can be tricky to diagnose because symptoms vary widely from person to person. Some people experience overwhelming fatigue; others feel out of sorts. Many individuals are keenly aware of their hopeless moods while others complain more about vague symptoms, such as feeling run-down or a lack of enthusiasm. The folks in the latter group commonly deny feeling depressed when asked. And sometimes a bad or sad mood is just a bad or sad mood.

In this chapter, you discover different types of depression and how to determine if SAD is a factor; we discuss a variety of things that can imitate SAD and point out the most dangerous side effect of any kind of depressive disorder or sadness: suicide.

Uncovering the Type of Mood Disorder

Mood disorders are, well, problems with your moods. SAD is actually a type of mood disorder, and to find out if you have a case of SAD, you first have to determine if you've ever had one of two specific types of mood disorders: major depressive disorder or bipolar disorder. If you suffer from depressive symptoms now or have in the past, we help you discover whether your problem is a major depressive disorder (what's also known as a clinical or unipolar depression) or bipolar disorder (a problem involving moods that fluctuate wildly). If you have one of these types of mood disorders and it comes and goes with the seasons, you may have SAD.

Exploring controversies with DSM

Just what is a mental disorder? Diagnosing an emotional problem doesn't come about with a simple chemical analysis or blood test. Psychiatrists, psychologists, and other mental health professionals typically refer to a document called the *Diagnostic and Statistical Manual (DSM)* for determining the criteria for any specific diagnosis of an emotional disorder. The reason professionals do so is to communicate with each other by using an agreed-on set of standards, which the DSM provides.

For example, the most recent revision of the DSM states that to have a diagnosis of major depressive disorder, you must suffer from depression for at least two weeks and experience five or more symptoms. Well, some people have only four symptoms, but the symptoms continue for 12 weeks or more. Does that mean that these folks don't have a major depressive disorder? That's one of the reasons the DSM is controversial; it isn't always clear if someone perfectly fits a given diagnosis.

Therefore, the DSM is constantly under revision and is considered imperfect in many ways. Professionals continue to disagree with aspects of the diagnostic criteria. Nevertheless, we employ the definitions from the DSM (in this book) when discussing mood disorders and SAD because they have the widest acceptance in the field.

However, you should know that Dr. Rosenthal (covered in the section, "Adding in the SAD effect"), who pioneered some of the research in SAD, prefers slightly different criteria for SAD. These distinctions are subtle and technical. We do agree with Dr. Rosenthal in one important respect. You can probably benefit from treatment for SAD even if your symptoms don't fit every single criterion on the DSM list.

On the other hand, some mood disorders don't come and go with the seasons and therefore aren't considered cases of SAD. Nevertheless, knowing and understanding your problems lay the foundation for your recovery.

Take a look at Jason's story:

> **Jason** puts the finishing touches on his master's thesis in economics. The project has consumed his time and thoughts for more than six months. He's confident that, once approved, his promotion at work is in the bag. Jason has looked forward to being a senior analyst at his investment firm since he began working a few years ago.

> Indeed, he receives a promotion a month later and finds the new job challenging. Jason feels like he's living a dream. He loves his Manhattan apartment and thinks that with his raise he can almost afford the rent. The young professional social scene in New York is exciting.

> Early in December, Jason comes down with a nasty cold. He feels unusual fatigue. He turns to donuts in the morning, a bag of chips from the vending machine midmorning, and a couple afternoon high-octane coffees to help him fight through the energy drain. But as his sniffles go away, his

lethargy lingers. He wastes away evenings and weekends in front of mindless television. His boss notices his lack of enthusiasm and plummeting productivity.

The holidays pass, and Jason checks in with his doctor. After a series of medical tests and appointments, he's diagnosed with depression. He works with a psychologist for a few months, and his symptoms improve. His energy returns and his work productivity soars. His psychologist dismisses him but warns him that he may have SAD, which can return next winter.

Jason's symptoms are characteristic of SAD, *and* they're signs of regular clinical depression. So what's the difference between the two? In this section, you review the various types of mood disorders.

Dealing with major depressive disorder

Major depressive disorder disrupts thoughts, feelings, activities, and your body. People suffering from major depressive disorder have thoughts that reflect hopelessness, pessimism, and low self-esteem. Accompanying feelings include guilt, regret, and profound sadness. Most people affected by this disorder withdraw from and lose interest in their usual activities. Their bodies typically respond with fatigue, appetite changes, and vague aches and pains.

Take a look at the items below — the signs and symptoms of depression. Check off those descriptions that you think may apply to you. Everyone experiences symptoms related to depression from time to time, but the symptoms usually clear quickly. However, if you experience more than one of these symptoms and they've continued for at least two weeks or more, you may be suffering from major depressive disorder.

❑ I basically feel like I'm worthless.

❑ Lately, I have more trouble concentrating.

❑ I think I'm a failure.

❑ My life is full of regrets.

❑ I can't seem to make decisions about anything.

❑ My life seems headed downhill, and I don't see things getting better.

❑ I'm not interested in the things I used to be.

❑ I get irritated about the smallest things.

❑ I feel guilty about how I've lived my life.

❑ Nothing seems like fun anymore.

❑ I feel empty inside.

❑ I find myself crying for no reason.

❑ I sleep too much.

❑ I can't fall asleep, and when I do, I wake up early in the morning.

❑ I feel overwhelming waves of sadness.

❑ I hate being around other people.

❑ I've gained weight and craved comfort foods.

❑ I don't feel like anyone really cares about me.

❑ My mood is miserable most of the time nowadays.

❑ I've lost my appetite and seem to be losing weight even though I'm not trying to.

The quiz is unlike many quizzes you've taken before because you don't pass or fail this one. This quiz gives you some indicators about your feelings and behaviors. In fact, checking *even one* of the above items can indicate a problem if it feels significant and/or is impacting your life in a major way. For example, if you only checked *I'm not interested in the things I used to be,* and you find yourself so disinterested in things that you have no motivation to work or go outside of the house, your symptom is causing you a real problem. And if you've checked more than three or four, your symptoms can be fairly serious. Either way, we recommend that you go see a mental health professional to determine the best course of action.

The signs and symptoms listed above are most often due to some form of depression. But physical problems can also mimic depressive symptoms. If you display these symptoms, we recommend that you see your family physician for a check up. Then you can consult a mental health professional if no physical basis for your difficulties is found. This book provides extremely useful help, but we don't generally recommend attempting to treat major depression entirely on your own.

Riding the rollercoaster of bipolar disorder

The term *bipolar* means having two poles. In the case of bipolar disorder, it means alternately experiencing two different, opposing states. This form of mood disorder, once known as manic-depressive disorder, usually involves alternating episodes of depression and mania. *Mania* is a state in which a person exhibits frenzied excitement and agitation.

The problem with calling this disorder "bipolar" is that the manic side isn't exactly the opposite of depression. Although mania involves euphoric feelings (which seem like the opposite of depression), it can also be a dangerous, frightening condition. On the other hand, you wouldn't call it mania if you're merely feeling the buzz from a triple latte with an extra shot of espresso. Nor if you found out that you just won the lottery — that's just what you call a really, really good day! Mania often starts out by you feeling pretty good, but then the behaviors start spiraling out of control.

Mania can be fairly mild and not cause severe problems, but it can lead to dangerous, even lethal behaviors and situations. For example, some people with mania become sexually involved with people they don't even know and fail to ask questions or use protection of any kind during sexual acts. Others seek wild thrills by driving at high speeds in dangerous places.

All degrees of bipolar disorder alternately involve depressive symptoms with some level of mania. The symptoms of mania include the following:

- ✔ A mood that's excited, elevated, and noticeably higher than normal
- ✔ Uncommon irritability
- ✔ Feelings of grandiosity ("I can do anything")
- ✔ Unusually poor judgment and decisions
- ✔ Feelings of substantial superiority over others
- ✔ Being much more talkative than usual — speech can also be quite rapid
- ✔ A significant reduction in the need for sleep as opposed to simply not sleeping well
- ✔ Rapidly jumping from one subject to another
- ✔ Taking excessive risks (gambling, sexual indiscretions, wild financial schemes)
- ✔ Feeling physically stirred up

Bipolar disorder is a serious mental condition. Although generally a chronic disorder, recent psychosocial and medical advances have made the disorder treatable and manageable. Please seek help if you or someone you care about show signs of mania. People with a severe case of bipolar disorder sometimes lose touch with reality.

Some professionals feel that bipolar disorder is a diagnosis that's overused and given without having a thorough diagnostic workup. If you're diagnosed with bipolar disorder, you may want a second opinion because the treatment of bipolar disorder usually involves medications with significant potential for side effects. We strongly suggest a second opinion if your child receives this diagnosis because long-term medication treatment may be required. See Chapter 6 for more information about medications for all types of depression.

Adding in the SAD effect

SAD is a type of a mood disorder that's a *specific* type of either major depressive disorder or bipolar disorder (for more info on these disorders, see the previous sections). SAD's distinctive feature is that the mood disorder has a *seasonal* component. Most typically, SAD symptoms start in the late fall and worsen in the winter.

Dr. Norman E. Rosenthal first investigated and popularized the phrase *seasonal affective disorder.* He grew up and received his medical training in South Africa and then moved to New York in the late 1970s to begin his psychiatric residency and research into mood disorders. The first winter after his move, he noticed as winter approached and nights got shorter, that his productivity and energy fell. As part of his research, he met with scientists studying biological rhythms and mood at the National Institute of Mental Health in Washington, D.C. His discussions with those scientists pioneered research into the causes and treatment of SAD.

Take a look at how Michelle starts to notice her SAD:

> **Michelle** belongs to an exclusive group of real estate agents in Seattle, Washington, known as the Prestige 50 Club. This membership consists of the top producing agents in the area. She exudes energy and infectious enthusiasm with her clients. She works hard, stays focused, and sells a lot of homes — that is for most of the year.
>
> Michelle usually finds that in the winter months, she has trouble motivating herself. She has less energy, typically puts on 10 or 15 pounds, sleeps more, and sells far fewer homes. Of course real estate usually slows down during the winter months, and Michelle attributes all her problems to that slowdown.
>
> However, this year her symptoms are beginning to severely impact her functioning at work. She oversleeps, misses appointments, neglects her clients, and makes careless errors on her closing papers. A close colleague suggests she may have SAD.

Although many of the signs of SAD are the same as for major depressive disorder or bipolar disorder, a number of them tend to be a little different from other types of depression. Like Michelle, you should look for the symptoms *particularly* characteristic of SAD:

- Carbohydrate cravings
- Decreased interest in sex
- Overwhelming fatigue

- Seasonal (fall and winter) occurrence, improving in the spring
- Sleeping more than usual
- Weight gain
- Withdrawal

Before most mental health professionals diagnose SAD, they have to see more than one episode of depression during the winter months. And sometimes among folks with bipolar disorder, manic episodes can emerge in the spring and summer, so professionals look out for that behavior as well.

Most researchers believe that SAD is related to the shorter days that accompany the arrival of winter months. Decreased daylight affects your body's internal clock (*circadian rhythms*) and chemistry. For more on circadian rhythms *and* the relationship between where you reside on this planet and your risk of coming down with SAD, head to Chapter 3.

In the realm of psychology, a field known as evolutionary psychology exists. This field involves the study of psychological phenomena that may have evolved as responses that improve adaptation to the world. Early humans who migrated away from temperate climates discovered that food supplies were more scarce in the winter. Therefore, some speculate that SAD may have been an adaptive response to the lack of food supplies. SAD often includes symptoms of low energy and slowed metabolism, which decrease the need for food intake. Interestingly, the most common symptoms of SAD sound a bit like a bear in the winter months. Bears prepare for winter by fattening up as much as they can. Their winter months are spent in hibernation, a period of time during which bears' metabolisms slow in order to conserve energy when their food supplies are scarce. They're inactive and withdrawn as compared to other times of the year.

Summer sad?

When you think of SAD, you may most commonly equate it with the season of winter. Winter SAD is by far the most common type of seasonally related depression, but much less is known about a type of SAD that occurs in the summer months. People who complain of summertime depression often cite humidity and heat as particularly troublesome for them. In contrast to people with winter SAD, summer SAD sufferers report more problems with a lack of sleep, poor appetite, and agitation.

Some people are more sensitive to changes in seasons and weather than others, which could make them more prone to either type of SAD. However, unlike winter SAD, summer-related SAD isn't likely caused by changes in amount of daylight (see more in Chapter 3).

Discerning What's Not SAD

SAD describes two types of mood disorders (major depressive disorder and bipolar disorder — see "Uncovering the Type of Mood Disorder" earlier in the chapter) that occur seasonally, most often in the winter months. But other types of mood disorders can be affected by the seasons. Check out the following sections to see if you're suffering from the seasonal blues.

Winter blues

The winter blues is similar to, but not as severe as, SAD. You may feel a little down for several days when it's overcast and cold outside, and that's not unusual. You're sludging through mushy snow and getting wet and cold and downright dirty at times (don't you just hate that sandy salt thrown all over the street and sidewalk?). But for most people, a nice cup of hot chocolate or a cheery fire is enough to perk up their moods until the sun comes out again. Symptoms that are pretty much the same as SAD, just less oppressive and usually fewer in number, persist throughout the winter season.

For example, people with winter blues become more fatigued, withdraw, and may crave carbohydrates. In addition, they usually sleep more than at other times of the year. (By the way, almost everyone we talked with in Alaska said they sleep more in the winter — even folks without the winter blues.)

Unlike people with full-blown SAD, some sufferers with the winter blues generally manage their lives okay during the winter. They go to work, attend school, and participate in activities, but they don't spring into these activities with much enthusiasm or interest (at least not as much as they do in the summer or spring). People with the winter blues meet most of their crucial obligations, but sometimes procrastinate more than usual, and their productivity usually drops.

The treatment for winter blues is much like SAD, but treatment is likely to work faster and more effectively. Unfortunately, most people with winter blues don't seek treatment because they think what they're experiencing is normal. But feeling consistently blah, lethargic, and down in the winter isn't normal or necessary.

Holiday blues

It's the most wonderful time of the year — but for some folks, that phrase is only a song and not a feeling. Many people report feeling painful sadness as they watch their friends engage in the holiday festivities.

While the winter holidays such as Thanksgiving, Christmas, Hanukkah, and New Year's can be prime triggers for holiday blues, any holiday can be a source of dread. The holiday blues occur just prior to, during, and sometimes for a short period of time following the holiday. Why, you may ask, is that the case — holidays are thought of as a time of celebration, right? Here's a list of reasons why some people suffer rather than celebrate the holidays:

✔ **Unmet, unrealistic expectations:** The holidays are full of high expectations for fun, entertainment, and downright dazzlement. Some folks go all out to prepare just the right food, decorations, and merriment. But if anything or anyone fails to live up to these lofty expectations, the person in charge collapses into a state of perceived failure.

✔ **Memories of loss:** Holidays are a time of reflection. These memories may be joyful, but for many people, holidays also trigger memories of loss through death, breakup, or circumstance. The contrast between the present day holiday and the past losses sometimes feels overwhelming. Compounding the problem is the fact that more people actually appear to die during the holidays than at other times of the year. Check out the nearby sidebar, "The holiday effect," for more information on why that could be the case.

✔ **The stress of the holidays:** Even if you don't participate in the decorations, gift giving, food gorging, cooking out, and various traditions of each of the holidays, stress increases for most people at those times of the year. Parking spaces disappear. Traffic increases. Crowds jam into stores, parks, or beaches. People often become irritable. The urge to spend too much money overtakes the best intentions of many to stay within a reasonable budget.

If you read about SAD earlier in this chapter (see "Adding in the SAD effect"), you may assume that people who have sadness during the holidays have a case of SAD, but they usually don't. SAD typically is more severe and lasts longer than the holiday season. If you think you're experiencing the holiday blues, but your low moods continue for more than two weeks, you very well may be experiencing a case of major depressive disorder or even SAD. Whenever such symptoms persevere, seek a consultation with a mental health professional or your family doctor.

To help break the cycle of the holiday blues, check out the following list of suggestions:

✔ **Eat and drink in moderation.** Alcohol makes you more depressed, and overeating triggers both sluggishness and guilt.

✔ **Do something for someone less fortunate.** Volunteer to serve the homeless on Thanksgiving Day or take extra blankets to a shelter or help collect toys for needy families.

✔ **Scale back your plans.** You don't have to be the big party planner and try to impress people. Attend some parties and don't be the host.

✔ **Reflect on the things you feel grateful for.** Make a list (see Chapter 19).

✔ **Don't spend too much money.** Make a realistic budget and stick with it!

✔ **Connect with friends and family.** Call someone you haven't seen in a long time. Invite friends over who may be spending the holidays alone.

✔ **Express difficult feelings with someone you trust.** If you're feeling down, talk it over with your partner, close friend, or mental health professional.

Chronic blahs

Dysthymic disorder is a type of depression that's like an unwelcome guest who comes to visit and then doesn't want to leave. The main difference between dysthymia and major depressive disorder is that dysthymia is milder but continues relentlessly, sometimes for years or even decades. People with dysthymia frequently fail to seek treatment and simply think that their condition reflects the way life is or part of their personality — kind of like winter or holiday blues (covered in the two previous sections) but persists all year long, year after year.

People with dysthymia display two or more of the following symptoms:

✔ Difficulty with making choices

✔ Fatigue

✔ Feeling hopeless

✔ Grouchiness and irritability

✔ Low moods

✔ Low self-esteem

✔ Pessimistic attitude

✔ Problems with appetite

✔ Problems with attention

✔ Sleep difficulties

Good news! Dysthymic disorder can be treated successfully. This condition isn't something you should just live with — because life doesn't have to be glum all the time. Most of the treatments for other types of depression can be successfully applied to dysthymia. Consult your doctor.

The holiday effect

It's bad enough that people frequently feel grief over the *past* loss of loved ones during the holidays, but surprisingly enough, researchers at the University of California, San Diego, and Tufts University School of Medicine, Boston, discovered that deaths occur in the United States at a higher rate on Christmas than any other time of the year and at the second highest rate on New Year's Day. And the spike in deaths on these holidays seems to have been increasing over the years.

The data suggests that a major cause of what the researchers called the "holiday effect" wasn't due to stress connected to the holidays, an increase in respiratory illnesses, or even over consumption of rich food or alcohol. Rather, it appears that people tend to delay going to urgent or emergency medical care on the holidays, which can then have fatal consequences.

Therefore, if you have serious medical symptoms of any type during the holidays, please seek medical attention with as much urgency as you would on any other day of the year! Whether you end up discovering your ailment is trivial or severe, we're pretty sure your family will be glad you're around to celebrate another holiday instead of mourning your loss at the next one.

Grief and loss

Grief is a normal reaction to many types of loss. People grieve the loss of significant relationships, friendships, and partners. However, people also experience grief in response to other types of losses:

- Appearance
- Health
- Income
- Job
- Physical abilities
- Status

Some of these losses occur at otherwise happy times, causing people to feel confused about their feelings of grief. For example, after looking forward to retirement for 40 years, some people feel unexpected grief at the loss of status, colleagues, and structure. Furthermore, normal aging can result in diminished physical capacities and changes in physical appearance and general health. All types of such losses and transitions can easily trigger grief reactions. When these losses occur in the winter months, especially around the holidays, they can weigh even heavier.

When you experience loss, you may feel sad, upset, and generally unbalanced. The emotional pain from some losses can be as intense as almost any physical pain. People frequently report difficulty sleeping, eating, and being happy. The more serious the loss (divorce or death), the more intense the pain.

Grief usually resolves gradually with time. However, grief sometimes endures at high intensities for a prolonged period. When grief doesn't slowly fade, treatment should be considered.

One major difference exists between grief and depression. Specifically, depressed people tend to harbor horrible feelings about themselves. They're self-critical and pessimistic. Although, those folks with grief feel sad, by contrast, their self-esteem doesn't suffer.

If you ever experience depressive symptoms without any apparent cause, you may want to consider whether you've suffered loss. And don't forget that seemingly happy transitions (kids growing up and leaving home, an exciting job change, graduation from college, and so on) can also involve significant loss. Any kind of change, positive or negative, can bring gains and losses.

Stress

"Adjustment disorder with depressed moods" is what psychologists say you experience when you respond to stress with sadness, tearfulness, depression, or hopelessness but not to the extent that you would with an episode of major depressive disorder. Adjustment disorders are connected to identifiable stressors, but they aren't unimportant. People with an adjustment disorder with depressed moods do experience some impairment in the way they function at work, school, or in how they relate with others. Some of these impairments include

- ✔ Difficulty concentrating
- ✔ Lack of enthusiasm
- ✔ Trouble making decisions

Just because your depression isn't considered major, doesn't mean you shouldn't seek help. If your low moods are disrupting your ability to perform to your usual standards, get help. Adjustment disorders typically are a little easier to treat (and possibly with less time) than other mood disturbances.

Losses pile up in the winter

The death rate tends to climb during the entire winter season in countries outside of the tropics. In particular, deaths increase from respiratory diseases and coronary/cerebral thrombosis (blocking of the arteries). One reason that respiratory infections increase is that people crowd together in more poorly ventilated areas. Cold air stimulates coughing and sneezing, which in turn spread infections more readily.

Strokes and heart attacks climb because of the way the body responds to cold. Blood flows away from the peripheral limbs and toward the core organs while it thickens at the same time. This process increases the risk of clotting and blocking of crucial arteries. Both of these risks are far greater to the elderly who are more vulnerable.

Diseases

Medicine agrees that specific diseases can contribute to or even cause depression. Furthermore, depression impacts the course of many diseases:

✔ More than 40 research studies found that heart attack patients who were also depressed or became depressed following their heart attack had a much higher risk of death.

✔ Many diseases lead to abnormalities in electrolytes, hormones, and endocrines that can directly cause depression.

✔ People who are depressed have lower white blood cells for fighting off infections, which is especially problematic for the elderly who already are at risk for impaired immunity.

✔ Diseases frequently cause losses due to incapacitation, stigma, and sense of identity — all of which can trigger depression.

✔ Depressed people tend to withdraw from relationships, but social support has been shown to reduce the risks of many physical ailments.

If you suffer from a serious illness, pay attention to signs of depression (for signs of depression see "Dealing with major depressive disorder," earlier in this chapter). Getting treatment for your depression may aid your recovery. Furthermore, if you're depressed and not getting treatment, your physical health may suffer.

Medications

Just as certain diseases may either worsen or cause depression, both prescription and over-the-counter (OTC) drugs used to treat a variety of ailments, can heighten or even cause depression, too. For example, a drug meant to sedate you or clear your sinuses, can make you feel lethargic, run down, and even depressed. Some drugs, such as hormones, may change the chemistry in your brain and thus produce depression.

A few of the more common prescription medications known to cause problems with depression include

- Anticonvulsants (for seizure and mood disorders)
- Benzodiazepines (for anxiety disorders)
- Beta blockers (for high blood pressure)
- Hormones (for birth control, menopausal symptoms, and so on)
- Interferon (for Hepatitis and cancer)
- Narcotics (for pain)

The list of medications that can cause depressive symptoms is quite long; the list above is merely an example. If you take any type of medication, whether prescribed or OTC, and have developed symptoms of depression, you should check with your doctor.

Guarding Against Suicide

Sometimes the symptoms of depression fade away within a few weeks with counseling or medication. But other times, depression, including SAD, is deep, dark, and persistent with the potential to become deadly. See the sidebar, "Shocking suicide statistics" if you want to know just how deadly depression can be.

In the meantime, look over the items in the following checklist, and check any that apply to you to determine if you're in need of immediate help.

- ❏ I often think about killing myself.
- ❏ I have planned a way to kill myself.
- ❏ I feel hopeless about the future.
- ❏ The world would be better off without me.
- ❏ I don't see any point in trying to get better.

❑ I tried to get help once, and it didn't work, so there's no point in going on.

❑ I can't envision a future for myself.

❑ I look forward to death.

❑ I feel completely unable to improve my situation.

❑ I have started abusing substances (drugs or alcohol) because I just don't care anymore.

❑ I don't even want to wake up in the morning.

If you checked even a single item above, please seek help *immediately.* If you can't wait for an appointment, call 911 and ask to be taken to an emergency room. You need to talk with a real, live person, whether that person is a physician or mental health professional.

In addition, consider the following contacts:

✔ **1-800-SUICIDE:** This number is staffed 24 hours a day, seven days a week with counselors.

✔ **1-800-999-9999:** The Covenant House Crisis Hotline's Nine Line is staffed 24 hours a day, seven days a week with counselors.

✔ **1-800-273-TALK:** This number routes you to the closest possible crisis center in your area.

✔ **www.befrienders.org:** Befrienders Worldwide provides emotional support and listens to people who are in distress.

✔ **www.who.int/mental_health/prevention/suicide:** The World Health Organization has a variety of information and sources about suicide.

If you worry that someone you love or care about may be suicidal, watch for the warning signs:

✔ Giving away valued possessions such as CD collections or a long-prized musical instrument

✔ Suddenly calling people he or she hasn't contacted in a long time, but makes no plan for continued contact

✔ Increased use of drugs or alcohol

✔ Getting in serious trouble in school or in the community (for example, a good student who totally ceases doing any schoolwork)

✔ Divorce or loss of relationship accompanied by other serious signs on this list or the previous checklist

✔ Dwelling on talk about dying (It's a myth that people who talk about suicide don't follow through)

Shocking suicide statistics

You may think that suicide is something pretty rare and that no one you know would ever follow through. The World Health Organization (WHO) recently reported that more people die from their own hand than die in wars and murders. Dentists, veterinarians, and doctors have access to lethal chemicals and are at particularly high risk. Pesticides are used in about a third of all suicides. In the year 2000, about 1 million people killed themselves around the world, and it's estimated that 20 to 60 million people made some kind of suicidal attempt. Suicide rates have increased by 60 percent in the last 45 years, and suicide now is among the leading causes of deaths of people from the age of 15 to 44.

If you have doubts about whether a person you know is contemplating suicide, talk to the person and ask. You won't implant an idea from out of the blue. If you think a suicide attempt is imminent, call 911. Let a professional help you figure out what's going on.

Chapter 3

Who Gets SAD and Why?

You may be reading this book because you think you may suffer from seasonal affective disorder (SAD) or you know someone who does. You may be wondering what your chances are of getting or having SAD. There are risk factors that can add up to the potential for experiencing SAD or winter blues. Just as with any emotional issue, some people are more prone to come down with SAD than others.

In this chapter, we outline the risk factors that play into SAD as well as how they impact the body's rhythms and cycles. Yes, you've got rhythm even if you can't keep time to the music! We also discuss how the body's chemistry and circuitry are involved, as well as look at some interesting research and share more actual case histories.

Recognizing the Risk Factors

Do you fit the typical patterns of those folks who have SAD? If you do, you still may never get it, and if you don't, you're not totally immune. We're talking about risk factors, not certainties. A *risk factor* is something about you that increases the likelihood that a certain outcome will occur. These factors include the following:

✔ Disturbances in your body's clock

✔ Living far away from the equator

✔ Not getting enough sunlight

- ✔ Recent move from the tropics
- ✔ Family history of depression
- ✔ Living in bad climates
- ✔ Being a female

Researchers remain somewhat unclear on exactly how important these risks are, and future studies are needed to clarify the relative contributions of each of these risks.

SAD is a treatable condition. Don't panic if you have a whole bunch of the risk factors above. You still may not develop SAD and you can do something about it if you do.

Some other risk factors do exist for developing SAD. Although they aren't necessarily the most significant contributors to SAD, they're important just the same.

Gender and hormones

Women seem to come down with SAD a little more often than men, although the reasons remain undetermined. Women may have a higher risk due to difference in their hormones. On the other hand, women tend to admit to feelings related to depression more readily than men, so women may be diagnosed more frequently with SAD than men simply because they're more open with their doctors about their feelings.

Researching temperature and moods

One problem scientists face in researching the effects of temperature on mood is that, in the industrialized world, most people spend the majority of their time indoors. So if you're shut in most of the time, weather and climate aren't going to affect you as much. However, researchers at the University of Michigan and a variety of other prestigious academic centers, conducted a series of studies that involved people spending varying amounts of time outside. These researchers found the following to be true:

- ✔ Moods improved with warmer temperatures when people spent more time outside in the spring.

- ✔ Moods deteriorate with hot temperatures when people spent more time outside in the summer.

- ✔ When temperatures were pleasant in springtime, people's moods worsened if they weren't allowed outside to enjoy the weather.

It's amazing how much time and money sometimes go into confirming the obvious. It's nice to be outside in the spring. But when you have to work inside while the weather's wonderful outside, it's a bummer. And when it's hot outside, it's not so great to have to spend much time out in the heat.

By contrast, men may go untreated for SAD because men often don't own up to having depression as easily as women do. According to researchers at the University of California-Davis, men complain more of irritability, minor physical ailments, and problems with concentration and focus as compared to acknowledging sadness or depressive feelings.

Age

SAD occurs more frequently among young and middle-aged adults. Although the risk is slightly less, children and adolescents can suffer from SAD. Depressive symptoms in the young are similar to depressive symptoms among adults. Young people report feelings of sadness, sleeping too little or too much, and changes in appetite. Other symptoms may include dropping grades, withdrawal from friends, and disinterest in usual school activities. People who are over 65 also have less risk for SAD.

Although it's good news that SAD occurs less frequently among the elderly, it appears that the rates of other forms of depression more than make up for that reduction. Between 6 and 9 percent of older folks have symptoms of a full-blown, major depression. However, as many as 10 to 25 percent of the elderly experience at least a few serious symptoms of depression. Sadly, almost half of the people in nursing homes appear to suffer from chronic depression.

Genetics

If you have family members who've been diagnosed with SAD or any other form of depression, your risk for SAD goes up. Genetics stands as the most likely reason for this risk factor, although the dynamics of one's family (for example, loss of a parent, abuse or neglect, and so on) may play a role as well.

Moods and weather

Climate and weather factors may impact your emotions and behavior. These factors include barometric pressure, humidity, temperature, and wind:

> ✔ **Barometric pressure:** Changes in barometric pressure foretell changes in the weather. When a storm is coming on, barometric pressure usually drops. The reverse is true as a weather system moves out of the area.

> A Canadian study found that acts of violence and increased emergency psychiatric visits surged during times of low barometric pressure. Apparently barometric pressure has some influence on aspects of brain chemistry that may account for these effects.

- **Humidity:** Humidity makes hot temperatures feel hotter and cold temperatures feel colder. Therefore, humidity likely affects moods as well. It doesn't take a rocket scientist to know that on hot, humid days people generally feel miserable. When it's cold and damp, it's also pretty hard to feel cheerful.

- **Temperature:** Extreme heat has been related to increases in irritability, anger, and violent crime. Some studies report that extremes in heat decrease your ability to remember things, slow your reaction time, and decrease mood. And as you get closer to the equator, the rate of summer related SAD increases (see Chapter 2).

  Extreme cold can also cause problems such as sluggishness, fatigue, and feelings of depression. Cold weather typically is associated with shorter days. So which is a greater risk factor for SAD, cold or amount of light one receives? The jury is still out on that one.

- **Wind:** Sitting on the beach in the sunshine with a gentle cooling breeze sounds like a pleasant experience, right? The wind can also blow away a good mood. Some scientists believe that the positive ions (see Chapter 8 for more details about positive and negative ions) created by winds cause negative effects on mood and thinking ability. Just ask anyone who lives in areas where dry winds whip through at certain times of the year. We just get irritable when a 40-mile an hour wind comes blowing through when we're trying to walk our dogs. That's not fun at all.

A tale from the south

There are far fewer cases of SAD as you approach the equator, and the cases are likely due to the weather (heat) and not a lack of light. But in the pursuit of science and our desire to leave no stone unturned, we decided that an expedition closer to the equator was in order.

The locals of Merida, Yucatan Mexico, claim that the gentle afternoon breeze has been arriving from the same direction for thousands of years. The weather and beauty of Merida — the Capital city of the Yucatan — is indeed astonishingly consistent. Aside from the occasional rainstorm or even rarer hurricane, this tropical city basks in sunshine pretty much year-round.

The people of Merida are noticeably warm and welcoming. Who wouldn't be though, with sunshine all year round? We know of no other researchers who've gone to Merida looking for SAD. We're proud to be the first. Upon arrival, we talked with almost everyone we ran across — our cab driver, the hotel clerks, university psychology faculty, and more than a couple of beverage servers. Yet for some reason we failed to find a single person who acknowledged having experienced SAD or even knowing of someone who had. *Were these people simply in denial?*

Probably not. You see, the average temperature in Merida ranges from a high of 85° Fahrenheit in May to a bitter cold high of 74° in January (or 23° to 29° Celsius). Well, the research wasn't exactly fruitful, but we did see some great Mayan ruins!

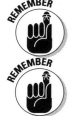

Because weather involves short-term fluctuations over hours and days, weather is more likely to affect short-term moods instead of causing a full-blown episode of SAD. Climate refers to long-term patterns and more readily induces long-term irritability or depression like that seen in SAD.

Summer-related SAD occurs more often in places where summer temperatures soar. You won't see SAD so much in the temperate tropics.

Feeling the Rhythm and Blues of SAD

The human body has rhythm — and we're not just talking about its ability to keep time to music. The body regulates most of its biological processes through various rhythms known as biological clocks. These processes include sleep and wakefulness, moods, hormone levels, menstrual cycles, eating cycles, temperature, pulse rate, metabolic rate, sexual drive, and so on.

The two most important rhythms for SAD sufferers appear to be circannual and circadian rhythms:

- ✔ **Circannual rhythms:** These rhythms occur over the course of a year and informs birds (in the Northern Hemisphere) when to fly south for the winter and return in the summer. Polar bears are active in the cold and spend the summer in torpor (a slumber like state). Other animals hunt and gather food in the spring, summer, and fall and hibernate in the winter.

  With humans, circannual rhythms aren't as obvious in their effects as with birds and polar bears. However, many scientists believe that circannual rhythms affect humans in areas such as weight gain and depressed moods in the winter and the opposite in the summer.

- ✔ **Circadian rhythms:** This cycle regulates your day/night clock. The word *circadian* comes from Latin and means *about or around a day*. Humans are diurnal, which means that they're active and working during the day, and they sleep at night (at least the majority of them).

  Your circadian rhythm is largely set by light. In general, darkness signals the body to slow down and prepare for sleep. Dawn stimulates an awakening process. As days shorten in the winter, your circadian rhythm tells you to go to sleep earlier and wake up later.

These natural rhythms have been affected by the advent of electric lights and alarm clocks as you see in the following section.

Hot tempers

Psychologists from the University of Missouri and Iowa State University looked at crime records for a 45-year period. They found that when days were hot, violence increased. In fact, in the United States, the hottest cities had more violent crime than the coolest cities. And the hottest years were associated with the most violent crimes. The authors also cited data indicting that major league baseball players get beaned by pitchers more often on hot days than cool days. Interestingly, property crime doesn't seem to go up or down with the temperature.

Clocks, circuitry, and chemistry

Before electricity, humans went to bed as daylight dimmed. For the most part, they went to sleep, and then got up when the sun rose. The body's clock was set by the sun rising and setting each day.

The body's clock has a location in the brain, and it's quite a mouthful. The location is called the *suprachiasmatic nucleus,* or SCN for short. The SCN is located in the hypothalamus (located below the thalamus near the middle of the base of the brain), which in turn regulates a wide variety of functions such as temperature, metabolic processes, sleeping, emotions, and even sexual feelings. The SCN receives information about the length of the day through the retina in the eye as it responds to changes in light.

As dawn approaches, your biological clock alerts your system to change the ingredients in the soup of chemicals that course through your brain and body. The SCN triggers an increased level of some chemicals and hormones while decreasing the production of others. The important mood-altering chemicals in your body include

- ✔ **Cortisol:** Cortisol stimulates alertness and gets you going in the morning. Cortisol increases energy and prepares you to meet the demands of the day. However, excessive cortisol can harm your health by raising blood pressure, contributing to obesity, and harming your immune system. In the morning, cortisol increases, and in the evening, it decreases.

- ✔ **Melatonin:** Melatonin is associated with drowsiness and a wide range of other effects on the body, not all of which are completely understood. See Chapter 8 for more information about melatonin. In the morning, melatonin decreases; in the evening, it increases.

- ✔ **Serotonin:** Serotonin influences a wide range of functions such as mood, temperature, sleep, memory, and appetite. In the morning, it increases, and in the evening, it decreases.

Disruptions in the levels and even the rhythms of the production of these hormones can have serious negative consequences for mood, energy, sleep, and health.

Months, seasons, and chemistry

Sometimes melatonin fluctuates across *seasons* (which is called a circannual rhythm) not just the day. Serotonin, an important chemical (technically called a neurotransmitter) that helps regulate mood, also has a seasonal and daily variation. In the winter, serotonin levels typically decrease for most people. People with SAD appear to be particularly sensitive to these decreases.

Interestingly, Canadian Drs. Lam and Levitt report that people with SAD demonstrate increased duration of melatonin production in the winter whereas people without SAD don't show a difference across the seasons. For people who *do not* suffer from SAD, normal indoor lighting may compensate for reductions in the amount of sunlight available in the winter. SAD sufferers, on the other hand, may require higher doses of light in order to keep their biological clocks and their melatonin production stable. See Chapter 5 for more information about the effects of light and SAD.

Stress, sickness, and chemistry

Many other things can also disturb your circadian rhythms. These factors include infections, toxic agents, life stressors, your coping ability, and even the way you think about things. Some researchers believe that disrupted circadian rhythms are an important contributor to all depressions; not just SAD.

The main difference between SAD and non-SAD depression may simply be that people with SAD are especially vulnerable to a lack of light in their environment. Check out Dennis' story:

> **Dennis** lives outside of San Diego, California, and works the day shift as a lab technician in the hospital emergency room. He amazes his friends and family with the clock that he seems to carry in his brain. He never wears a watch or sets an alarm clock. He wakes every morning within two minutes of 5:00 a.m. — every single day, even on the weekend. If you ask him the time, he can tell you with an accuracy of two minutes or less. Dennis leads a somewhat regimented life. He likes routines and punctuality.
>
> Dennis really hates the traffic he fights everyday because it makes his commute unpredictable. In fact, last winter, he fell into a depression and assumed it was triggered by his disdain of snarled traffic. So he jumped at

the chance to switch to a schedule at work called a rotating shift. This shift requires Dennis to work 12-hour stints, all of which start and end outside the usual congested traffic patterns. However, these shifts change around every two weeks.

Suddenly, the clock in Dennis' brain went on the fritz. His accuracy at knowing the time slipped by five or ten minutes, and soon, he started waking up at odd times and needed to buy an alarm clock. He suffers from insomnia for the first time in his life. His irritability has increased, and he developed road rage even with the reduced traffic. He's feeling lethargic and tired most of the time. Everything seems out of whack.

His mood worsens as the fall days shorten, even though he lives in sunny San Diego. He starts thinking about quitting his job. Dennis slips into a full-blown case of SAD. This episode far exceeds the depth of his first depression. The combination of shorter days and the disruption of his normal day/night cycle throw his body's rhythms into utter chaos.

 If you struggle with adjusting to changes in daily routines, try to keep your schedule as regular as possible. Go to bed at close to the same time each night; eat at regular intervals; and when circumstances interfere with your routines, plan some down time to relax and rejuvenate.

Locating the Latitude in Your Attitude

Do you remember Geography in grade school? If so, perhaps you recall the lesson that introduced the imaginary lines that circle our globe. These lines are called latitudes (or parallels because they run parallel to each other). You probably recall that the circle spanning the middle of our earth is called the equator. The equator has a latitude of zero. Successive circles become smaller as they approach the north and south poles. Generally, the further you're located from the equator, the greater your risk for SAD.

 Latitudes are assigned numbers (designated as degrees) that describe their distance from the equator. They range from 0 to 90 degrees north at the north pole and 90 degrees south at the south pole. Latitude lines are spaced about 69 miles apart. The larger the number, the further they lie from the equator. So a latitude of 10 degrees would be approximately 690 miles from the equator. In actuality, the distance varies a little because the earth isn't a perfectly shaped sphere.

Light and latitude

In the Northern Hemisphere the earth tilts somewhat closer toward the sun in the summer, and this tilt creates longer periods of daylight. The further from the equator you go, the longer the days. In the winter, the northern part of the earth tilts further away from the sun and results in shorter days and longer nights.

Where humans went (and go) wrong

The earliest humans appear to have evolved in areas near the equator. Close to the equator, the amount of sunlight remains fairly constant throughout the year. Basically, you get 12 hours of daylight and 12 hours of darkness every day, all year long. These early humans had biological clocks based on these evenly spaced days and nights. These clocks told them to hunt and be active during the day and to rest, sleep, and recuperate during the night.

A variety of occurrences in the ensuing thousands of years have probably caused disruptions in some people's circadian rhythms:

✔ People migrated further away from the equator, which resulted in great variations in the length of days and nights in winter and summer.

✔ In general, people spend far more time inside, away from natural lighting. Electric lights provided a substitute for the sun. Such lights appear to have different effects on people's circadian rhythms. Sufferers from SAD seem to need more than standard indoor lighting to regulate their circadian rhythms.

✔ Long distance travel creates jet lag, which involves a temporary, but significant disturbance in the body's clock.

✔ Life becomes more complex and stressful. Work invades home life through 24/7 available cell phones, faxes, and instant messages. These invasions may throw off your body's rhythm.

✔ Shift work is common in certain occupations and often runs completely counter to regular day/night cycles.

Some individuals seem particularly sensitive to disruptions in their circadian rhythms. Pay attention to whether your body has difficulty making adjustments to disturbances in routines such as travel across time zones, changing work schedules, or interruptions in sleep.

The opposite occurs in the Southern Hemisphere. Winter falls during the months of June, July, and August, and the days are shorter and the nights longer. Summer comes during the months of December, January, and February.

To keep things simple, we refer to the seasons instead of the months when we talk about SAD.

Most research suggests that SAD occurs far more frequently in the winter when days are especially short and people are exposed to less sunlight. Hundreds of studies examine the relationship between increased latitude and the incidence of SAD. Although some exceptions exist, in general, the risk for SAD increases as you go further away from the equator.

However, other factors such as cloudy weather, pollution, and the length of twilight and dusk (when the sun is just below the horizon) also enter into the picture. Twilight and dusk are much longer in the far northern and southern latitudes. In fact, in regions above 60°24' N and below 60°24' S there is at least one night in which some sunlight is present in the sky a full 24 hours.

In the Northern Hemisphere, the longest day of the year is called the summer solstice, which generally occurs about June 21st or 22nd. In the Southern Hemisphere, that day would be called the winter solstice because it's the shortest day of the year down there. The winter solstice in the Northern Hemisphere occurs around December 21st or 22nd.

Even if you've never suffered from SAD your entire life, relocating to a latitude further away from the equator can trigger the onset of SAD:

> **Hannah,** a successful physician recruiter for a south Florida hospital, tears open the envelope from King's College Hospital in London. As she quickly scans the letter, she grabs her cell phone and speed dials her sister, Heather. "I got the job!" she excitedly tells her Heather, "I'm headed to England, I start work August 15th!"

> Hannah moves to London. She finds a flat and quickly makes friends with her coworkers. She loves her work and England truly feels like home. By the end of September, she phones Heather and relates that's she's never been happier in her life.

> Just a few weeks later Hannah notices that she's having trouble getting up in the morning despite sleeping well and going to bed at her usual time. She stops indulging in fish and chips after realizing her clothes are getting tighter. Hannah begins spending more time alone and loses interest in socializing. By the holiday season, she finds herself crying for no reason, and her mood darkens. She's mystified because she doesn't recall ever feeling like this before. She's always been upbeat, cheerful, and optimistic.

> Her sister, out of concern, flies to London thinking Hannah may be homesick. Heather's worry grows as her sister fails to be cheered up by her visit. Heather convinces Hannah to see a doctor who explains that a move from a southern climate to a northern climate can sometimes trigger an episode of SAD. Heather and Hannah feel better just knowing there's a name for what Hannah has probably been going through.

SAD and latitude quirks

The further away from the equator, the shorter the daylight in the winter. The darker the days, the higher the risk for symptoms of SAD. Even people who don't experience full-blown SAD are a little more likely to sleep more, eat more, have less energy, and feel down.

So, if you live in Florida you're less likely to develop a case of SAD than if you live in Fairbanks, Alaska. In fact, residents of Fairbanks run as much as a 25 percent risk of developing SAD whereas the risk for Floridians runs far lower. Seems pretty straightforward, doesn't it?

Perplexing issues with latitude and attitude

Even though latitude appears to affect the overall rate of SAD, some studies have actually failed to find a relationship between latitude and SAD. One of the problems researchers face is that they use the same instrument (test) to measure SAD across all cultures. Sounds like a good idea; however, when you translate these tests, the meaning of the questions can change quite a lot.

Research is a slow, complicated process, and it takes numerous studies before a clear picture begins to emerge. For example, in some eastern countries, they have relatively few words for describing depression. And symptoms of depression seem to vary somewhat from one culture to another. So any single study you may read can be misleading. SAD research is much like research in many other arenas. That's why one day you may read in your morning paper that coffee greatly increases your chances of dying from heart disease. You then vow to stop drinking coffee, but then two weeks of caffeine withdrawal later, you read that coffee is basically good for you.

Alas, the issue of latitude isn't simple and neither is the risk of developing SAD. Getting SAD isn't just about living in darker, colder places far away from the equator. Different studies suggest that in some areas of the world SAD rates are much lower than you may expect given their latitudinal locations.

For example, people in Iceland (where it can get pretty darn cold and dark in the winter), don't appear to suffer much from SAD. Scientists think that their lower rate of SAD may be because Icelandic families have lived there for a very long time — thousands of years actually — and therefore may have developed genetic adaptations to the darker winter seasons. As a matter of fact, when people from Iceland migrate to Canada, they remain somewhat immune to developing SAD while their Canadian counterparts suffer from relatively high rates of SAD.

Culture enters into the SAD picture in important ways too. Northern Norway is actually in the Arctic Circle, and if latitude was the only thing going on, Norwegians would suffer from very high rates of SAD. But they don't. In the long, dark days of winter, people in Norway celebrate with various special social activities. Numerous festivals celebrate the arts, the nights, and the northern lights. Abundant candles brighten homes and offices. Norwegians attempt to create a warm, bright, environment indoors in contrast to the stark, cold, and dark outdoors.

When you travel to China or Japan, the situation gets even murkier. The rates of SAD in those countries are much lower than in the United States. One study indicated that summer SAD (which is relatively rare in the Western Hemisphere) is actually more common among the Chinese population than winter SAD. See Chapter 2 for a more thorough discussion of summer SAD.

So what do all these findings mean about the relationship between SAD, latitude, and the amount of light people are exposed to during various seasons? Read the sidebar on "Perplexing issues with latitude and attitude" if you want to know more. But the bottom line is that latitude and light usually do influence whether you're at risk for SAD.

Tales from the north

Alaska in the early autumn is a time of contrasts. The weather can range from glorious to ghastly. So in the interest of science, we decided to take a field trip to Alaska. The changing trees glistened in the sunshine; the rivers and lakes sparkled. We hiked through glorious meadows red with fire weed and through golden stands of trees. In the distance the mountains were white-blue with glaciers. How can anyone be depressed?

Interestingly, most of the people spoke of SAD as a disorder that others had. But in the next few sections, you read some stories of Alaskans with SAD. Their stories capture the essence of what other Alaskans told us.

Making it through the dark days

Admitting to weakness or vulnerability just isn't something Alaskans do easily. Luther, in the story that follows, doesn't usually like to talk about himself, especially when it concerns his feelings. His story demonstrates how SAD can affect even the robust and hardy folks:

> **Luther** starts preparations for winter in the early fall. He makes sure he has enough fuel to keep the house warm and food, so when the inevitable storms rage, his family can survive. He reports that in the beginning of the dark season, he feels invigorated, almost excited. He enjoys gathering the wood, shopping for supplies, and making sure the vehicles are maintained. It's early in September, and he already has chopped six cords of wood (a *cord* is a lot of wood).

> Luther's voice drops when he talks about the dark season. He says that sometimes the wind doesn't stop, and the temperature doesn't climb as high as zero for weeks. He begrudgingly admits that his mood typically darkens with the decreasing light. By January and February when spring seems like it will never arrive, he finds himself in an abyss.

> Luther eats more, sleeps excessively, and drinks too much. He and his wife argue more during the winter, and evenings are often spent in sullen silence. Like many Alaskans, Luther carries a rifle to protect himself from errant elk — over time he's become rather enraged by what he considers to be one of the world's stupidest animals. He admits that his irritability has increased over the past few years and is much worse during the winter.

Luther has never told anyone about his feelings and is surprised to hear what SAD is and that it's treatable. He says that he's heard about light boxes but as far as he's concerned, those things are hogwash.

Seeking help for SAD

Some people don't develop SAD immediately after moving north. Linda in the example below demonstrates how SAD can strike after living in the same place for a number of years.

Linda moved to Alaska about 20 years ago. She was a teacher and heard about the great pay and job opportunities in education in Alaska. Linda recalls the excitement of her first winter in the north. She filled her small home with warm quilts, candles, and bright lights. It helped that she had just started a relationship with the man she eventually married. However, after several winters, Linda began to have problems. It didn't occur to her that she may have SAD and attributed her overwhelming fatigue to the changes she'd experienced. During the course of a few years Linda married, had two children, and advanced in her career.

She had a breakdown during the sixth winter after she'd arrived in Alaska. She couldn't seem to get out of bed and had bouts of crying. She finally went to her physician who started her on an antidepressant medication. She now takes her medication a few weeks before the light changes and tapers off during the spring (see Chapter 6 for more information about medications for SAD).

"I love living here. I view SAD like having a cold. You try to prevent it, but when you get one, you take good care of yourself. If the symptoms get really bad, you seek professional help."

Getting too much of a good thing

Jennifer is an example of someone who found herself overly stimulated by the effects of excessive amounts of daylight.

Jennifer grew up in Anchorage, Alaska, but she attended college in southern California and graduated with a degree in business. Although Jennifer enjoys the California weather, she's anxious to return to her home. The Barrows, Alaska, branch of an energy company eagerly recruits her not only because of her academic standing, but also because she's lived through the Alaskan winters without having problems. The company has experienced considerable turnover in its entry-level staff because of the harsh climate.

Jennifer begins her job in August, after taking a few weeks to rest and move following her graduation. She finds the work difficult and the 40-hour weeks challenging. The nights are longer in Barrows than in Anchorage, but she doesn't really mind the months of darkness. The fall turns to winter, and she realizes that her adjustment to the northern climate has been fairly painless.

As spring approaches, she feels her mood begin to soar. The sun doesn't set for 82 days in Barrows, Alaska. There are no trees in Barrows, but she doesn't really mind. She's a bit more concerned that the nearest Big Mac is to be found 425 miles to the south in Fairbanks.

Nonetheless, she finds herself anxious to start planting a garden. She joins an evening softball league and increases her social activities. She volunteers for extra projects at work and expects that she'll get a promotion before the end of her first year.

She notices as the days lengthen that she's having a hard time sleeping. By early May, the constant daylight is beginning to annoy her. She buys blackout curtains, but that doesn't seem to help. Her thoughts seem to be racing and she finds herself irritable. She attributes it to lack of sleep. She heard that taping aluminum foil to her windows may help, but it doesn't seem to improve her sleep.

Just as too much darkness can affect mood, as seen in the example above, constant daylight can upset the circadian rhythm as well. Some people suffer from insomnia, hyperactivity, racing thoughts, and feelings of irritability. Although not too common, a few people actually have what's called a hypomanic or manic episode.

If you find yourself not sleeping; your mind seems to race; you feel irritable; you start spending too much money or make risky plans; you just may be experiencing an episode of mania (see Chapter 2 for more information). Contact your physician or a mental health professional for an evaluation. Although mania can actually feel terrific, it's a dangerous condition. Fortunately, most people with SAD don't experience mania.

Chapter 4

Getting Help for SAD

* *

In This Chapter

▶ Deciding on self-help or professional assistance

▶ Looking through the self-help options

▶ Navigating the professional maze

▶ Evaluating the fit with your professional help

* *

*I*f you suffer from seasonal affective disorder (SAD), you have options for treatment. Some people do well on their own through *self-help*. Others prefer or need to enlist the direct support of a professional. Even those folks who seek help also employ some level of self-help under the direction of a therapist (a copilot of sorts). How you determine the best source of help or what you call your flight plan depends on how serious your SAD is as well as other factors discussed in this chapter.

This chapter offers a quiz to help you decide if you can go it alone or would be better off enlisting some help (check out "Figuring Out If You Need a Copilot"). If you can fly alone, you get some guidance on which direction to go. But if you determine that you can use some help, you also find descriptions of the types of professionals (*copilots* as we like to call them) who can work with you, a list of questions to ask to help select the right person to help, and tips on how to ensure a smooth flight.

Determining the Help You Need

We're believers in self-help. After all, we've authored a half dozen or so self-help books. And a considerable body of research on self-help indicates that it works for many people. But we also work as clinical psychologists and know full well that some people need or simply prefer professional assistance.

Check out this section and see whether you're a candidate for self-help, professional help, or a combination of the two.

Going it alone

Self-help involves finding your own solutions to problems. Solutions don't come out of the clear blue sky. The key to self-help is that you research answers on your own. A great place to start is with self-help books such as this one (also see Appendix B). You can also conduct your own research at the library or on the Internet. After you find your remedies, you put them into practice.

Characteristics of a solo flyer include having relatively mild symptoms, enjoying research and reading, and feeling comfortable working independently. Here's an illustration of someone who may be fine treating SAD on her own:

> **Kelly** lived in Minneapolis, Minnesota, last year and was diagnosed with depression. She attributed it to her stress while finishing her master's degree in biology. This year she moved to Manitoba, Canada, to take a research job at the local university. She describes herself as an independent outdoors adventurer. She looks forward to cross-country skiing and her new home.
>
> Toward the end of October, Kelly notices her mood deteriorating once again. One of her colleagues tells her about SAD. That evening Kelly goes home and searches the Internet for information. She recognizes that her symptoms fit those of SAD, although they aren't as severe as some people's. Kelly orders a couple of books and vows to get outside more, buy a bright light box (see Chapter 5), and work through the exercises in *Seasonal Affective Disorder For Dummies*. By late November, her mood has improved substantially. She feels hopeful and upbeat.

Kelly is a good candidate for self-help. Her symptoms aren't severe and her motivation is still pretty high. She enjoys research and is an avid reader, so her self-help techniques meshed with the things that she liked to do in her life.

Asking for help

Characteristics of someone who would do best with a copilot include having fairly severe symptoms (see Chapter 2), feeling overwhelmed, and preferring to work collaboratively with others as opposed to alone. Here's an example of someone who needs a copilot:

> **Kevin's** seasonal depressions consistently appear each November and fade by April. This year, Kevin's SAD hit especially hard. He missed three days of work, and his boss wrote him up for absenteeism. When he does manage to show up to work, Kevin can't concentrate or get anything done. Kevin feels like giving up.

A co-worker suggests that Kevin read *Seasonal Affective Disorder For Dummies*. Kevin picks up the book, but can't get past page six. He just can't seem to find the motivation to do much of anything.

Right now, Kevin isn't a great candidate for going solo. His symptoms are too severe to expect that self-help alone will suffice. He needs the support and advice of a trained mental health professional. As his treatment proceeds, he may very well find the book he purchased quite helpful — as an addition to his therapy.

Figuring Out if You Need a Copilot

Some people really like to do things on their own, and others like the idea of working on a team. One approach isn't better than the other. However, sometimes getting help makes a whole lot of sense.

If you're uncertain about whether you need professional help or if you can work through your SAD on your own, take a look at Table 4-1 to figure out which plan of action may best suit you. This quiz is simple; just check *yes* or *no* to each question.

Table 4-1		Determining Your Flight Plan Quiz
Yes	***No***	***Question***
		1. I've been missing work due to my depression.
		2. I enjoy researching issues of interest to me.
		3. I've been feeling suicidal.
		4. I prefer to work on projects by myself.
		5. I feel utterly hopeless.
		6. I'm an independent learner.
		7. I've been abusing drugs (legal or illegal) or alcohol.
		8. I've a track record of getting things done.
		9. I'm not meeting my usual obligations.
		10. I can muster at least a reasonable amount of motivation.
		11. I'm making really bad decisions lately.
		12. I like to read nonfiction sometimes.

If you checked yes on *any* of the odd-numbered questions, consider seeking professional assistance. The odd-numbered questions are signs that your depression is fairly serious and impacting your life in a major way.

The more even-number questions you answered with yes, the more likely you would make a good candidate for self-help (again, assuming you didn't answer yes to odd-numbered questions). If you didn't answer yes to any of the even-numbered questions, you still can benefit from self-help, but you may prefer to combine it with help from a professional.

The remainder of this chapter helps you see the options for either going solo or seeking help with a copilot. All of the chapters in this book can be used for reference purposes in self-help endeavors or in conjunction with a professional.

There's no absolute, definitive way to determine who succeeds through self-help alone. But if you're a good candidate from the quiz, feel free to try flying solo. If your flight gets choppy, or off course, get a copilot (see "Choosing a Copilot" later in this chapter).

Finding Self-Help Options for SAD

The word *self-help* seems to be a little off in meaning because support groups involve other people, just as choosing to turn to family and friends do. So, even though you choose the options for self-help treatment, going this route doesn't mean it has to be a lonely trip.

Self-help for SAD comes in several forms, but the options are more limited than they are for depression in general. However, most good resources for other types of depression can be applied to SAD. Here are the most common approaches:

- ✔ **Books:** You probably know about this option because you're reading this book. Advantages of this strategy include the fact that books are fairly inexpensive, and if you own the book, you can go back and reread sections as needed and take notes in the margins. Good self-help books usually tell you what the research has shown in any particular area. Check out Appendix B for other good book suggestions (we usually suggest that people read several books on the topic).

- ✔ **Family and friends:** When depressed, people typically pull away from family and friends. They hunker down and isolate themselves. All too often in those cases, family and friends feel rejected. This perceived rejection sometimes leads friends to stop making contact with people who have SAD. So instead, stop the cycle of isolation and make contact with both your family and friends.

Although we heartily recommend increased contact with your loved ones, don't turn to them for therapy. Even professional psychologists make lousy therapists for their own families. That's because they care too much and are too close to their loved ones to be objective.

✔ **Web sites:** You can find substantial information about SAD at various Web sites (some listed in Appendix B). Many research institutes and universities have sponsored Web sites that provide accurate, scientifically based advice.

Be cautious and check out the credibility of your sources. If the site offers what sound like "miracle cures" or expensive products, take extra care. If you're not sure, ask a licensed health professional for an opinion.

✔ **Self-help groups:** Support groups help you feel connected and often have good ideas for how to cope. You may have to work a little to find self-help support groups for SAD in your area (unless you live in the United Kingdom where they have a group called the Seasonal Affective Disorder Association [see also www.sada.org.uk]). However, a wide variety of support groups exist for major depressive disorder or bipolar disorder (see Chapter 2), and you may find these groups useful as well.

✔ **Chat rooms:** We wouldn't have written about chat rooms ten years ago, but today you can find them on almost any imaginable topic, including SAD. People log on and post questions, comments, suggestions, ideas, and experiences. Sometimes people feel a connection like they get with support groups without having to leave their homes.

Chat rooms and self-help groups at times can get overly negative. The focus sometimes turns to how horrible things are instead of what can be done to resolve your issues. If that starts to happen speak up and try to take the group in a different, positive direction. Quit the group if it isn't productive and meeting your needs. Everyone needs to complain sometimes; just don't let it get out of hand. Finally, you don't know who's participating in chat rooms so be careful about revealing personally identifying information.

Choosing a Copilot

The decision to seek help is a courageous one and doesn't in any way signify weakness. But knowing where to turn can feel a tad daunting. A lot of people are confused by the array of professionals in the mental health field. They ask, "What's the difference between a psychologist and a psychiatrist?" "What's a counselor and how is that different from a psychotherapist?" "Should I just go to my physician or nurse practitioner for help?"

Ethical practice in mental health

No matter which professional you choose to work with, licensed mental health professionals adhere to a fairly consistent set of ethical standards. Although each profession's standards vary a little from each other, they have much in common. General principles include the edict to do no harm. In other words, professionals strive to improve the lives of their clients while respecting and protecting civil and human rights. They're also trained to maintain confidentiality in regard to your personal information. But you need to know about the few exceptions to that confidentiality rule. These exceptions include

✔ If you reveal intent to seriously harm yourself or someone else

✔ If you disclose that you or someone you know is abusing a child or elder

Some insurance companies may also require disclosure of information (which is why some people prefer not to use their insurance for mental health purposes).

Dual relationships are also prohibited by most ethical codes. These relationships include romantic or sexual relationships between a therapist and a patient. They also include certain types of business transactions between therapists and their patients. Most therapists provide information about these ethical guidelines and the nature of the therapy relationship in a document called an Informed Consent prior to you starting therapy. If your therapist doesn't do so, ask about these issues.

This decision is a very important one, and it's not a bad idea to ask for help. Here are a few places to turn when you need advice on seeking a professional mental health provider:

✔ One place to turn for advice is your family doctor. Doctors are often the first person people go to, and they usually know good, local mental health providers.

✔ If you plan to use your insurance, your insurance company may have a list for you, too.

✔ You can also call your local university psychology or counseling department.

✔ Don't forget to check with friends, especially if you know someone who has worked with a therapist.

✔ You may also want to check with your priest or pastor.

✔ You can check with professional associations for each type of mental health provider.

Be sure to take notes when you ask providers about their backgrounds. Here are a few good questions to ask:

✔ **Are you licensed to provide mental health services in this state?** After you determine the type of license, verify the answer on the Internet. If the answer is no, find someone else who is.

✔ **What are your fees?** Fees vary widely and sometimes are even negotiable. Check with several providers and compare, although price is only one factor out of many to consider.

✔ **Do you take insurance?** Some good practitioners don't take insurance so be sure to ask if it's important to you. Without insurance, you spend more money out of your pocket.

✔ **What hours do you see people?** Depending on your work hours, you may need to be seen in the evenings or on weekends.

✔ **Are you familiar with treating SAD?** Some highly qualified mental health practitioners have no experience with SAD. We recommend that you only consider going to someone who has training and experience in the treatment of SAD.

✔ **Do you employ therapies that have been validated by scientific research?** Not all licensed professionals have been trained in approaches that have been scrutinized by research studies. Some of those approaches may work, but it makes sense to seek therapies that have been shown to be effective by a number of studies. The primary treatments known to be effective include the following:

- Cognitive-behavioral approaches (see Chapters 9, 10, 14, 15, and 16)

- Light therapy (see Chapter 5)

- Medications (see Chapter 6)

Just so you won't be totally in the dark sorting through titles, degrees, and expertise within the mental health profession, the following sections offer definitions for those pros you're most likely to bump into.

Primary care health practitioners

Primary care health practitioners are trained in treating a wide range of medical problems. Physicians, nurse practitioners, and physician assistants generally fill this role. This source is a good place to start because these providers can assess whether your emotional symptoms that look like SAD actually have a physical basis to them.

Some of these health practitioners are also trained in *mental health* issues, but that their experience in this field varies greatly. Even if they haven't had such training, they usually know good mental health professionals to refer you to.

The majority of medications for SAD are prescribed by these professionals (see Chapter 6 for more information on who prescribes medications for SAD). However, when medication issues are complex, your primary care provider may refer you to a psychiatrist (see the next section).

Psychiatrists

Psychiatrists are physicians who've also received advanced training in the diagnosis and treatment of emotional disorders, including SAD. Following medical school, psychiatrists typically complete a four-year residency program in psychiatry. Most psychiatrists emphasize and are experts in biological treatments such as medication (see Chapter 6) and electroconvulsive therapy (see Chapter 8). Therefore, they're more likely to prescribe medication instead of psychotherapy. However, psychiatrists vary greatly in their training and interest in psychotherapy. Therefore, check with any particular psychiatrist to see what approach that person takes and to see if that approach matches your interests.

Social workers

Social workers have a master's degree in social work and supervised training in psychotherapy. If they deliver mental health services in the private sector, they need to have a license in the state in which they practice.

Social workers are usually well trained in the diagnosis and treatment of emotional disorders such as SAD. They don't prescribe medications, and they aren't referred to as a doctor. Social workers usually have special expertise in finding social services and governmental assistance.

Clinical and counseling psychologists

Clinical and counseling psychologists hold a doctorate degree in clinical or counseling psychology (either a PhD or PsyD). In addition to the advanced degree, these psychologists must complete a one-year internship followed by a one- to two-year postdoctoral training program. Clinical and counseling psychologists are experts in the science of human behavior, diagnosis, and treatment of emotional and behavioral disorders. Psychologists frequently specialize in the delivery of scientifically validated psychotherapies (not all psychotherapy has been found to be effective in research studies).

Counselors and psychotherapists

You can find many well-trained individuals who are licensed by the state in which they practice to provide diagnosis and treatment of emotional disorders. Most licensed counselors and psychotherapists have a master's degree in psychology, theology, counseling, or a closely related field. Typically, these professionals also have some period of supervised practice prior to obtaining their license to work independently.

Other people with signs on their doors

A lot of people claim expertise in providing mental health services and activities that sound something like psychotherapy. The range of such services includes listening to sounds on earphones, being hypnotized, exploring past lives, low-level magnets, energy fields, and so on (see Chapter 8 for alternative therapies). It's nearly impossible for the typical consumer to know which of the widely varying approaches may actually have some promise.

Many of the people providing these services aren't licensed by the state in any way. Some may even have ads with initials after their name, but for the life of us, we have no idea what the initials stand for! If you're tempted to try a therapeutic approach that's not discussed in this book, please check it out with a licensed mental health practitioner. Sometimes slick unlicensed "therapists" can be quite charming and flattering. You may even get a temporary lift from seeing them. But you can easily spend a lot of money on worthless therapies.

If you've previewed the various types of licensed mental health providers (covered in the previous few sections), start making calls and gathering facts. Don't be afraid to ask questions — you have a right to receive good answers. Any service provider who hesitates to answer, who fails to return phone calls, or who provides questionable information, should be avoided.

Keeping Your Flight Smooth

Whether you decide to go solo or choose to have a copilot, you still need to evaluate how things are going with the choice you've made. If you go solo and don't make good progress or your symptoms worsen, you may want to seek additional, professional help. And if you choose a copilot, you may discover at a certain point that you no longer need professional assistance and can continue improving on your own.

Assessing your self-direction

If you choose to go it alone, carefully monitor how things are going. Your moods should start improving within a month or so. You should feel reasonably optimistic that things will continue getting better. If you have trouble getting up in the morning or getting yourself to do the exercises recommended in this book, you may need to enlist a copilot like Melinda:

> **Melinda** begins taking yoga and reading about SAD. She quickly notices an improvement in her moods. She loses a few pounds and feels her energy rising. Unfortunately, a sprained ankle from a slip on the ice causes her to stop going to yoga for a while. Her moods promptly plummet. She decides to talk to her doctor about finding professional help.

Assessing your copilot

You've chosen a copilot and have started your trip toward overcoming SAD. Great! But what if the flight gets a little bumpy? How do you know if you experience normal turbulence or if you go off course?

Any therapeutic relationship takes a little time to develop. And you very well may feel a little discomfort at times, especially in the first four or five sessions. Nevertheless, sometimes people just don't click. If you aren't improving or you feel uneasy, you may need to find a new copilot. And that's okay!

A good therapeutic relationship contains two primary components:

- ✔ **Communication** involves an exchange of ideas, thoughts, and information.
- ✔ **Relating** refers to the emotional connection between you and your therapist.

Just because your therapist has a degree doesn't mean that she's a good match for you. Nor does it tell you if the communication and relating are working as they should. The next two sections give you guidelines for evaluating if your therapist is a good fit for you.

Can we talk?

The first component of a good therapy relationship is good communication. Therapy isn't likely to go anywhere without open, honest talk. Good communication includes these elements:

- ✔ **Do I feel comfortable saying almost anything to my therapist?** This comfort may take several sessions to develop, and that's okay because trust can take a while to evolve. But by the fourth or fifth session, you need to feel you can say whatever you want.

- ✔ **Do I feel my therapist truly hears what I have to say?** If you bring up a concern about your relationships at work and your therapist is a little dismissive of your issue, that's not a good sign.

- ✔ **Does my therapist talk clearly and not use too much professional jargon?** Occasionally professionals use terms to convey a meaning that's important. But they also need to explain such terms to you in words you can understand.

- ✔ **If my therapist says something I don't understand, do I feel free to ask questions?** In a good therapeutic relationship, you feel comfortable asking for clarifications or explanations about almost anything, and these explanations are given freely.

- ✔ **Does my therapist give me clear answers to any questions I have?** Sometimes the answer may actually be, "I don't know the answer," but all answers at least need to be understandable.

Anytime you seek professional services, whether for your finances, health, mental health, or your automobile, you need to be able to evaluate how well the relationship is going. If you don't feel that good communication is present, strongly consider changing your service provider.

Not that into you?

The second component of a good therapeutic relationship is the connection between you and your therapist. It's important that you feel accepted and understood. Your therapist should appear caring and concerned. Again, this connection can take a half dozen or so sessions to emerge. But if it doesn't, discuss the issue and consider changing therapists if you don't feel good about the answers.

- ✔ **Does my therapist seem genuinely interested in my issues?** Ideally you know that your therapist is interested by her questions and facial expressions. On the other hand, if she consistently seems distracted, that's not a particularly welcoming sign.

- ✔ **Does my therapist seem reasonably warm as opposed to cold and distant?** The answer to this question is somewhat subjective, but you need to feel cared about. On the other hand, this connection doesn't mean excessive warmth and affection or friendship outside of the therapeutic relationship.

- ✔ **Does my therapist seem nonjudgmental and uncritical?** It's okay if your therapist disagrees with you about an issue. But that disagreement shouldn't take the form of criticism or harsh judgment. For example, many therapists want their clients to do activities between sessions in order to speed up their recovery. However, if you don't do the "homework," therapists shouldn't scold or criticize you. Good therapists understand the difficulties in carrying out their advice.

✔ **Does my therapist get defensive?** When you ask for clarification or if you question or challenge the therapist's opinions, does she respond with irritation or anger or put you down in some way?

✔ **Does my therapy feel collaborative?** Good therapy feels like a partnership or an alliance. You need to feel that you're on the same page.

✔ **Does my therapist help me figure out goals and ways of accomplishing them?** Few people have the time and money to undertake years and years of therapy. Therefore, you get more done if your therapist helps you define the purpose of therapy and both short- and long-term objectives.

✔ **Does your therapist lecture you or guide you?** Lecturing, or being told what to do, has its place. But most people don't like to be told what to do. Don't you like to think that you've figured it out all by yourself? In fact, solutions worked through on your own, with a little guidance, are more effective than trying to apply what you've been told to do. The best copilots don't fly the plane for you (lecture); they help you figure out how to fly on your own.

Lecturing therapist

This example is a therapist *lecturing* a client about sleeping too much — a common problem for people with SAD:

Client: I've been sleeping an incredible amount, but I still feel like I'm not getting enough.

Therapist: Look, you've got SAD. And that often makes people sleep too much. I think that's what you're doing. You need to start getting up whether you feel like it or not.

Client: Yeah, but it's so hard.

Therapist: Yes, it is, but it's what you have to do.

Client: How come I feel like I *need* more sleep? I think I might not make it through the day.

Therapist: You don't really need more sleep; it just feels that way. Start getting up by 7:00 a.m. no matter what.

How does this example make you feel? If you were in the client's shoes, would you feel belittled and criticized? In the example above, the therapist fails to hear the client adequately and shows almost no empathy. Instead, she argues and lectures.

Guiding therapist

Another example shows a therapist dealing with the issue of sleeping too much (same issue from the previous section) in a *guiding* way:

> **Client:** I've been sleeping an incredible amount, but I still feel like I'm not getting enough.
>
> **Therapist:** How long has this been going on?
>
> **Client:** Oh, I guess ever since the end of October.
>
> **Therapist:** And when did you start getting depressed?
>
> **Client:** About the same time. Do you think it's part of my SAD?
>
> **Therapist:** Probably, that would be a common symptom. Is it okay for you to sleep that much or is it getting in your way?
>
> **Client:** Well, it's been hard for me to get to work on time, and I'm not getting enough things done during the day.
>
> **Therapist:** Do you think there's anything you may be able to do about this problem?
>
> **Client:** Well, I could get one of those dawn simulators I read about. That might help.
>
> **Therapist:** Great idea.

How does this example make you feel? If you read the previous section ("Lecturing therapist"), the guiding style feels more affirming and empowering, doesn't it? The client came up with a good solution, and the therapist simply guided him to it.

Good therapists help you figure out when you're ready to decrease sessions and/or terminate. At that point you use the tools you discovered in therapy on your own. And if you ever experience symptoms again, you can always go back to therapy for a while.

Part II
Examining the Biological Treatments for SAD

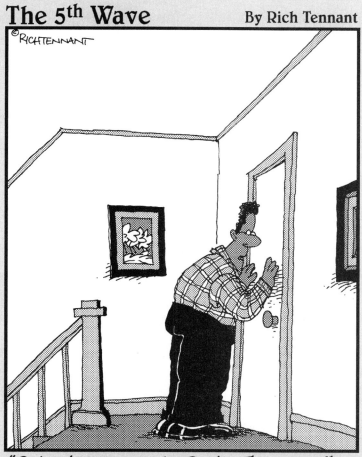

"Only six more weeks Doris. The groundhog saw his shadow. Do you need more chips or soda?"

In this part . . .

In Part II, we review the biological-based treatments for seasonal affective disorder (SAD) and begin illuminating the first treatment specifically designed to treat SAD — light therapy. You also start discovering the various medications for SAD and decide whether you want to talk to your doctor about that approach.

People with SAD often have food cravings, and to help you battle the bulge, we give you useful advice on managing your diet while you suffer from SAD. If you think you may want to use alternative treatments for your SAD, you get the lowdown on those in this part, too!

Chapter 5

Shining Light on SAD

● ●

In This Chapter

▶ Lightening up your moods

▶ Figuring out if light therapy is for you

▶ Getting help to turn on the lights

▶ Brightening up with light therapy

● ●

Seasonal affective disorder (SAD) is a type of depression that researchers believe is related to the dark dreary days and nights of winter. In general, those folks who live further away from the equator are more prone to SAD because of decreased sunlight in the winter. The shorter days beginning in the fall start the SAD symptoms, and the lengthening days in the springtime bring relief.

Much like a warm fire on a cold night cheers you up, increasing the intensity of light in your life may help lift your moods. Light therapy was conceived as a means for addressing the deficiencies in light that contribute to the development of SAD (see Chapter 3). In this chapter, you discover the ins and outs of light therapy — the first treatment that was specifically designed for SAD. You decide if light therapy is for you and how to design your own personal light therapy plan.

Good Morning Sunshine!

Most people report feeling a tad more lethargic around the winter solstice — the darkest days of the year. For people with SAD, symptoms are more severe and interfere with their everyday functioning, such as getting up on time, eating a healthy diet, and being productive at work. Common SAD symptoms include eating too much, sleeping too much, and feelings of sadness (see Chapter 2 for more info about symptoms of SAD).

Scientists in the late 1980s, particularly Dr. Norman Rosenthal, thought about the connection of decreased sunlight and winter depression. They hypothesized that if there was a way to increase the amount of light a person suffering from SAD was exposed to, then maybe the SAD symptoms would improve. They were right. Today, many studies confirm that light therapy can reduce the depressive symptoms of SAD. So, how does it work? The example below illuminates the point.

> **Amanda** was diagnosed with SAD while in college and was successfully treated with medication. She now works as a mechanical engineer in Milwaukee, Wisconsin. This fall has been particularly harsh, cold, and cloudy. Amanda leaves her heated garage before 7:00 a.m. and drives to work in the dark. She parks in a covered garage adjacent to her lab. By 5:00 p.m. when she gets off work, it's already getting dark, and she usually heads straight home.
>
> In early November, she begins to feel more fatigue; she craves high-carbohydrate foods, and starts to feel dreary. She recalls that her doctor warned her about her high risk of relapse (see Chapter 17). Therefore, last year, she and her doctor came up with some ideas on how Amanda can respond to an increase in SAD symptoms.
>
> Amanda remembers that SAD is thought to be caused by a lack of light in the winter. Amanda realizes that she needs to take action before her symptoms get worse. So, she decides that she needs more light in her life.
>
> Packed away in her garage is a purchase she made last year. It's a light box that emits 10,000 lux (see "Wishing you good lux" later in the chapter). She sets up the light box on a table next to her reading chair. She decides to set aside 30 minutes each morning to sit in front of her light box while reading the paper.
>
> After a few days of light therapy, Amanda feels better. She has more energy, and her cravings have decreased. She knows that her thinking is much more optimistic, and she believes that she can survive the winter and beat her SAD.

Sounds pretty easy. Turn on a light. Feel better, sleep better, maybe even lose some weight. Alas, there's a little more to light therapy than that. Check out "Deciding to Lighten Up" to see if light therapy may be an approach to try.

Deciding to Lighten Up

Light therapy is a safe and effective treatment for many people with SAD. You can potentially brighten your mood, give yourself more energy, and decrease food cravings by turning on a bright light. Sounds like a no-brainer. However, light therapy isn't for everyone.

Take the quiz in Table 5-1 and see if this treatment may be for you.

Table 5-1		Bringing More Light into Your Life
Yes	**No**	**Question**
		1. I've checked with my doctor or mental healthcare professional and have been diagnosed with SAD.
		2. My schedule is fairly regular. I get up and go to bed at about the same time each day.
		3. I can plan on spending 30 minutes or more each morning sitting in front of a light box.
		4. I've checked with my doctor about any medications that I might be taking that could cause photosensitivity.
		5. If I have eye problems such as retinal disease, diabetes-related problems, or macular degeneration, I've checked with an ophthalmologist before choosing light therapy.
		6. I don't feel irritable or edgy when I sit in bright light.
		7. I don't suffer from headaches or nausea after sitting in bright light.
		8. If I have a history of skin cancer or lupus, I've consulted with my doctor and gotten the go ahead.

So how did you do? If you answered *yes* to almost all the questions above, then light therapy *may* be an appropriate treatment for you. You should find a professional who has experience in this area to help you along the way and answer any questions that come up. If your primary care doctor doesn't know about light therapy, ask for a referral to see a specialist.

A *yes* response to questions 4, 5, and 8 of the quiz is especially important if you're considering light therapy. Although most professionals consider the risks to be fairly low, be sure to discuss these conditions with your doctor before starting light therapy. See "The Dark Side of Light Therapy" in this chapter for more cautions.

If you merely suffer from a case of the winter blues (see Chapter 2 for information about the winter blues), you could probably undertake light therapy without professional consultation (other than the issues in items 4, 5, and 8 of the quiz). But if you experience side effects, either stop the therapy or get consultation.

SAD is a type of mood disorder and can involve serious symptoms including the desire to hurt yourself, serious problems with concentration, and more rarely, very illogical thinking. For that reason, you should consult with a professional for help monitoring your progress and to address any undesirable side effects associated with light therapy. If you've been diagnosed with bipolar disorder or manic depressive disorder (see Chapter 2), you shouldn't try light therapy without close supervision from your healthcare provider.

The Nuts and Bolts of Light Therapy

So before you go out and buy a light box, you may want to know if it really works. The answer to that question is both yes and no. In other words, research says that light therapy works *very well* for many people, and some people don't seem to benefit much at all. Unfortunately, you can't know ahead of time who benefits and who doesn't.

The upside of light therapy is that it isn't terribly expensive (see "Figuring out Costs and Insurance" later in this chapter), and if lights are going to work for you, they'll likely do so fairly rapidly. Furthermore, you probably won't get nasty side effects from light therapy, but if you do get side effects, they're usually fairly mild.

If you want to pursue light therapy, it isn't as simple as flipping on a switch. You need to consider quite a few issues. In this section, we walk you through them.

Wishing you good lux

Light is described in terms of intensity or illumination. The technical term for the measure of intensity is *lux*. Here are some sources of light and the amount of lux (intensity) that they emit:

- Most living rooms in the evening: 300 lux
- Typical office: 400 lux
- Cloudy day outside: 3,000 lux
- Sunny day outside: 10,000 lux
- Really bright, sunny day: 100,000 lux

So, how many lux do you need? Most experts agree that light therapy treatment requires between 2,500 and 10,000 lux. If you're going to take this route, you might as well purchase lights that emit about 10,000 lux because light boxes that emit fewer lux typically require more time to work as effectively.

News flash: Rats and light

In 2006, *Behavioural Brain Research* reported a study in which scientists kept sand rats in a cage. The cage was bright for five hours each day and dark for 19 hours. This procedure lasted for three weeks. Another group of rats hung out in a 12-hour light/dark cycle, much like the day/night cycle that exists near the equator.

Then the scientists put the rats in a pool of water where they had to sink or swim. The rats from the darker homes sank faster, so the scientists concluded that sinking was a sign of depression. So the take-home message: Don't go swimming if you have a bad case of SAD!

Timing is everything

Bright light therapy involves a number of issues that all relate to timing. These issues include the length of exposure, the time of day you use the lights, and the times of the year you start and end the therapy. Timing takes experimentation and a willingness to be a little flexible.

How much time does light therapy take?

Most people benefit from exposure to bright lights for about 30 minutes a day (although there's not a hard and fast rule). However, some people reportedly require as much as two hours per day, and a few folks seem to get by on as little as 15 minutes. Therefore, you may need to experiment in order to find the right amount of exposure for you.

Here's how to get started:

1. **Start with 30 minutes of light exposure per day for a week or two.**

2. **If your symptoms don't start improving, consider increasing your exposure by 15-minute increments.**

   If you get up to two hours of light exposure each day, increasing further isn't likely to help you. Don't despair; if light therapy of up to two hours per day for ten days or more doesn't help you, other effective treatments are available. We describe these treatments throughout this book as well as help you decide if you may need professional assistance (see Chapter 4).

What time of day do I turn the lights on?

A majority of people with SAD find that exposure to bright light therapy works best in the morning — so turn your light box on in the morning. Generally, the earlier in the morning, you turn the box on, the better. That's because of the way light therapy seems to affect your circadian rhythms (see Chapter 3 for more info about circadian rhythms). In fact, if you move your light therapy from 7:30 a.m. to 6:00 a.m., you may fall asleep earlier in the evening and wake up earlier in the morning.

Artificial light and SAD

Melatonin is the hormone produced by the body in response to darkness. (See Chapters 3 and 8 for more information about melatonin.) Most people produce about the same amount of melatonin for about the same length of time each day in all four seasons. However, for people with SAD, melatonin secretion occurs for a longer period of time through the day during the winter, especially in areas far away from the equator. Dr. Wehr and colleagues wondered why.

The researchers asked non-SAD suffering volunteers to subject themselves to a month of 14-hour-long periods of darkness — similar to a northern winter but *without the benefit of artificial lighting* that most people have in their homes. They were also asked to spend the same amount of time in an environment with eight-hour periods of darkness — similar to a southern summer.

In this study, these non-SAD volunteers demonstrated the same kind of fluctuations in melatonin secretion that occur in SAD sufferers. The researchers speculated that most people's brains interpret artificial light as the equivalent of sunlight. However, SAD suffers may require more intense lighting to keep the duration of melatonin secretion constant across the seasons.

So if you have SAD, this research indicates that you need more intense light than other people in order to keep your melatonin levels and your body rhythms working like they should.

On the other hand, a few people seem to do better with getting their light therapy in the early evening. However, light therapy late at night can disrupt your sleep cycle.

With a little fiddling around, you can find what works best for you. Just make your changes slowly. See the section "If Lights Aren't Brightening Your Moods" later in this chapter for information about altering your light plan when it doesn't work right away.

What time of year should I try light therapy?

If you've already been diagnosed with a current episode of SAD, start your light therapy now! If you've suffered from several episodes of SAD in the past, you may want to start your bright light therapy a week or two before you tend to experience symptoms. Continue light therapy until spring or around the time you've previously recovered.

Some people put off their bright-light therapy until they get SAD symptoms. Those folks tend to have rapid recovery once their therapy has started; however, the longer you wait, the greater the chance that you experience depression for longer than you want. Because light therapy is safe and typically involves few side effects, avoiding depression altogether seems like a reasonable approach.

Types of lights

With regard to bright light products, safety comes first. If you are making your purchase in the United States, look for light boxes that are approved by the Underwriter's Laboratory (UL). In Great Britain or Europe, they have a safety mark called the S mark that indicates the device has been reviewed for safety standards. Other countries have various safety codes that are equivalent. Just make sure that your product has been evaluated by a recognized safety standards organization.

After you've considered safety issues, you can choose from a variety of products. The next sections show you your options.

Fluorescent lights in a box

Most bright light boxes contain a set of fluorescent lights in a box with a plastic diffuser. You want to buy one that's been rated at 10,000 lux of intensity because boxes with lower ratings require longer exposures to be effective. Also, be sure that your light box has a filter for UV rays. UV rays can damage your eyes and increase your risk of skin cancer.

Manufacturers and distributors of light boxes often promote the value of "full spectrum" light boxes for bright light therapy. However, most research has shown that the extra expense of such lights doesn't provide extra therapeutic benefit, so why waste your money? Not only that but also full-spectrum lights actually contain more UV rays, which you don't want.

If you're a handy person and think you want to make your own fluorescent light box, you can do that if you want to. But be sure you know what you're doing! It's easy to make an unsafe product. We know what would happen if we tried to manufacture our own light box (the risk of it burning down our house is a scary image), so recommending this approach is difficult!

LED lights

Light emitting diode (LED) lights last far longer than standard incandescent or even fluorescent lights (see preceding section). How much longer you ask? Apparently, LED lights can be used for 100,000 hours before losing about half of their intensity (more than ten years of continuous use!). They stay cool and emit no harmful UV rays.

Currently, insufficient research doesn't support the effectiveness of LED lights for SAD — not meaning that they don't work; it's just that they're pretty new on the market. However, the odds are good that they *will* prove to work as well. There's simply no logical reason why these lights wouldn't work at least as well as fluorescent lights. Some investigators believe that LED's emitting blue light may ultimately prove to be more effective than white light because blue light excites the eye more. However, this increased effectiveness remains unproven at this time.

Babies and light

The effects of lighting on sleep have been studied in newborn babies. In the past, if you visited a Neonatal Intensive Care Unit at a hospital, you were greeted by bright, constant lighting throughout the day and night. Although some hospitals still maintain such lighting, more modern facilities are changing that practice.

Science Daily recently reported that hospitals such as Vanderbilt's Children's Hospital in Nashville, Tennessee, are providing lighting that mimics natural day/night cycles. Studies have found that this cyclical lighting causes infants to sleep through the night sooner than if the babies had received constant lighting. They also appear to gain weight and generally thrive better in these cyclical conditions. The upshot of these studies is that they highlight once again the intricate relationship between light and biological processes.

Dawn simulators

In the winter, dawn comes later in the morning which may increase your difficulty in awakening. A dawn simulator is a light that gradually increases light output at a pre-set time. You set it to begin slowly brightening your bedroom up to two hours before dawn. Even while you're still sleeping, you are being exposed to increased light.

Several studies indicate that dawn simulators decrease SAD symptoms. Researchers speculate that simulators work by resetting your body's circadian rhythms (see Chapter 3 for more information about circadian rhythms and SAD). The brightness of dawn simulators tends to be much less than for typical bright light therapy with either fluorescent or LED lights.

Visors

An effective, but slightly odd looking, way of delivering light therapy is the light visor. Picture a baseball cap with lights mounted underneath the visor. Theoretically, you can deliver increased lighting to the wearer of the cap for many hours each day with little inconvenience.

You can wear the hats just about anywhere — on airplanes, driving a car, or at the office. Of course, you may have to put up with some jokes, and many people just may not understand your apparel. Besides that, there isn't a great deal of evidence concerning the effectiveness of visor lighting. Simply put, more research is needed on this one.

Enhancing Therapy with Helpful Hints

Successful light therapy depends on motivation. And the more convenient and pleasant you make your time spent receiving bright lights, the more likely you can keep motivated.

The biggest impediment to getting better with light therapy is that people simply don't do it. In fact, research shows that approximately half of people who try light therapy discontinue using it. Yet, people buy their light boxes enthusiastically and with good intentions. But, like the lonely treadmill in the garage or the unused gym membership, they don't give lights the time and effort that are required.

So, keep the lights shining in your home with some bright ideas:

- ✔ **Make a cozy comfortable therapy area.** Light therapy takes considerable time. If you sit on a hard, uncomfortable chair, you may stop therapy prematurely. Some people choose to set up a light box in front of stationary exercise machines so that they can accomplish two goals at once.

- ✔ **Have something to keep you occupied.** Most people need about 30 minutes a day to benefit from light therapy. You can read, watch television, talk on the phone, exercise, or eat as long as you look in the general direction (not directly at it!) of the light box. (The only time we find ourselves wanting to stare blankly for 30 minutes without doing anything is when a book deadline is approaching. Hmm, seems like a good idea right now.)

- ✔ **Sit close enough to your light source for maximum benefit.** Read the manufacturer's recommendation for the best distance. In general, the brighter the light, the further you can be from it. A foot or two distance is typical.

- ✔ **Set a regular therapy time.** During the day sit in front of your lights and make the time a priority. The more routine the therapy is, the easier it will be to keep it up.

- ✔ **Develop regular sleeping patterns.** Light therapy may help regulate your sleep patterns. But still, wake up and go to sleep at about the same time each day. Depression can worsen with fatigue. See Chapter 13 for more information about sleep.

- ✔ **Get help and advice.** Seek assistance from an experienced professional if you don't feel better in a couple of weeks. SAD can be a complicated problem. You may need a little help in tweaking your light therapy. And there are other types of help available, so don't give up.

The Dark Side of Light Therapy

For most people bright light therapy is safe and effective. But sometimes annoying side effects can occur. The following list provides you with the most common problems and what to do about them:

- **Trouble sleeping:** A few people who use light therapy develop insomnia. This problem can usually be addressed by sitting in front of the lights earlier in the day. If that doesn't work, shorten the time that you spend under the lights in 15-minute increments.

- **Agitation:** This issue can be a troubling side effect. People with this side effect report feeling stirred up or hyper. Very rarely agitation can signal the beginning of a manic state (see Chapter 2 for more info on mania). If decreasing the amount of light doesn't stop these feelings, seek immediate consultation with a professional.

- **Eyestrain or irritation:** Permanent damage to the eye hasn't been a reported effect of bright light therapy. Nevertheless, if you experience discomfort, decrease the time and intensity of your treatment and consult your doctor. Usually this discomfort can be managed by starting bright light therapy at around 30 minutes per day and gradually increasing the dose 15 minutes each day.

- **Feeling sick to your stomach:** Some people have bouts of nausea that tend to diminish over time. This side effect occurs in people who respond well to light therapy. So, don't give up immediately if you feel slightly sick. Again, the best way to respond is by decreasing exposure by 15 minutes per day until the feeling passes.

- **Darkening or redness of the skin:** If your light box is filtering out all the UV rays, this side effect shouldn't occur. However, some people with very sensitive skin may be affected. Light therapy appears to work through the retina instead of the skin. So, using sunscreen is a good idea that should solve the problem and not affect your treatment. As with all side effects, don't hesitate to contact your healthcare professional with concerns.

To ensure a safe experience with your light therapy, check out three more cautions:

- Don't use a sunlamp or a tanning lamp for light therapy. These products put out dangerous levels of ultraviolet (UV) rays. UV rays have been associated with the development of skin cancers. Therefore, therapeutic light boxes should have filters for UV rays.

 ✔ If you have a history of skin cancer, any type of skin disease, or extremely sensitive skin, be sure to consult a dermatologist prior to starting light therapy, even if your lights have the recommended UV filter. The same advice holds for eye problems, except that you should consult an ophthalmologist.

 ✔ With whatever type of light you use, don't stare directly at the light source — eye damage can occur. You should position yourself to look in the general direction of the light and/or the surfaces the light illuminates.

Treating other disorders with light therapy

SAD is the topic of this book, but people with SAD often have other problems. You may find it interesting to know that light therapy has shown intriguing possibilities for helping with such other difficulties:

✔ **Being a night owl:** Some people have trouble falling asleep at night and waking up in the morning. "Night owls" prefer to stay up very late at night and wake up very late in the morning. There doesn't seem to be a problem with that except when you have a 9-to-5 job.

Solution: If you're the night owl type and stay up late, try light therapy and/or dawn simulation therapy early in the morning. This procedure shifts your sleep rhythm so you can fall asleep sooner in the evening and wake up earlier in the morning.

✔ **Being a rooster:** "Roosters" fall asleep very early at night and get up at dawn or even a little prior to sunrise. No problems seem to exist unless there's a mismatch between your biological rhythms and your obligations.

Solution: If you're a rooster and fall asleep and wake up too early, you can try light therapy in the early evening. Doing so shifts your sleep cycle to a later time.

✔ **Eating, drinking, and smoking:** Some preliminary studies suggest the possibility that light therapy might provide a little boost in your efforts to overcome these problems, especially if your moods seem heavily influenced by the seasons.

We question light therapy for these issues, so if you struggle with substance abuse or eating disorders, please get professional help *first*. Light therapy might be tried as an additional tool, but you're likely to need more.

✔ **Other types of depression:** If you have a depression that doesn't seem related to the seasons, you may assume that light therapy wouldn't be for you. But adding light to your life actually might help. A few studies have indicated that bright light therapy works for depression unrelated to the seasons (see Chapter 2 for more info about other types of depression). However, it doesn't appear to add much to the effectiveness of medication if you're already taking an antidepressant.

Other tips? Turn on the lights; brighten up your home; enjoy the sun streaming through a window; take a walk in the sun. Ancient cultures worshipped the sun for a reason. You know intuitively that sunshine warms and heals the heart.

Combining Lights with Other Treatments

If light therapy works, then why would you need to consider another form of treatment? Well, some people who use light therapy don't fully recover from SAD. Therefore, adding another treatment makes sense. And frankly, many people eventually get restless or bored sitting in front of a light box. Then they become inconsistent or even discontinue light therapy prematurely. When that happens, SAD symptoms quickly return. Therefore, some people prefer alternative or combination therapies.

Studies that look specifically at the benefits of combining light therapy with other forms of treatment for SAD haven't been completed, so, we really don't know for sure that the combination works better. But other treatments described in this book can successfully decrease or eliminate SAD symptoms. Treatments include

- ✔ **Medication:** Clinicians found that people who use light therapy probably require lower doses of medication than people who don't. We tell you about the pros and cons of medication in Chapter 6. If you're successful with light therapy, you're likely to benefit from medication.

- ✔ **Cognitive and behavior therapy:** The outcomes are excellent for people who participate in cognitive and behavioral therapies (see Chapters 9, 10, 14, 15, and 16). The benefits of these therapies include no negative side effects and a decrease chance of relapse.

Any of these approaches can be easily combined with the others.

If Lights Aren't Brightening Your Moods

You could purchase a light box and dutifully sit near it for 30 minutes a day and discover that the world feels as dark as ever. So if light therapy isn't helping your moods, before you give up, consider a few issues and options covered in this section.

Start earlier

Start your light therapy in the early morning. If that doesn't work, try making it 30 minutes earlier. If you still don't benefit, you may consider using your lights in the early evening. However, make your changes in light therapy one at a time for at least ten days to two weeks, because if you change the intensity and the time of day you use the light box all at one time, you won't know which change was important.

Go outside

Consider taking more walks outside. Outside light on a sunny day is much brighter than light from a box. Of course, walking outside has a few dark sides to it. In higher latitudes, daylight doesn't occur until later in the day in the winter, sometimes much later, depending on how far north or south of the equator you live. And most people find that they benefit most from light exposure early in the morning.

Furthermore, many days in the winter are cloudy, and the amount of light is less than most light boxes. And then there's the fact that you probably don't walk staring at the sky and if you do, you may trip over a rock and hurt your-self (and then we aren't going to cover your hospital bills). So if you walk out-side and look at the ground, you may not actually receive that much extra light. Finally, sometimes walking outside in the winter on especially windy or cold days, can be a little daunting.

See Chapter 14 for more information about the benefits of going outside for light, and Chapter 15 for information on how exercise impacts mood.

Brighten your home and/or workplace

In addition to your bright light box, consider boosting the output of light in your home or work setting. Here are some suggestions:

- ✔ Buy higher wattage incandescent bulbs
- ✔ Buy more lamps
- ✔ Add additional indirect lighting
- ✔ Paint your walls a lighter color to reflect more light

However, we do *not* recommend white carpeting — that was one of the stu-pidest things we ever did in our lives! White furniture seems like an equally bad idea, but then that's just our opinion. We have two dogs that like romping in the mud and running madly around the house. We've tried to explain to them to wipe their paws before coming in, but they just aren't catching on.

Figuring Out Costs and Insurance

Light therapy is relatively inexpensive when compared to other treatments like medication or psychotherapy. You may need to take medications throughout the winter months for many years or forever. The costs of psy-chotherapy are reduced somewhat by the fact that you may not need to con-tinue it much beyond your first round of perhaps 20 sessions or so.

Bright light and work ethic

Do you ever get tired in the afternoon? You come back from lunch, sit down at your desk, start to yawn, and desperately wish you could take a nap. Researchers in Tokyo, Japan, studied the effect of light on afternoon sleepiness. They assigned normal workers to one of three groups:

✔ **The nap group:** This one sounds best to us. These lucky folks got to take a nap for 20 minutes after lunch.

✔ **The light group:** These folks worked near a bright window.

✔ **The dim group:** This group worked in 100 lux light, which isn't very bright (see "Wishing you good lux," earlier in the chapter).

Before and after receiving their specific intervention, the researchers administered tests that measured participants' drowsiness. One of the tests was called the Karolinska Drowsiness Test. (We know you don't need to know the name of the test, but we thought it was a funny name.) The researchers concluded that exposure to bright light through the window worked better than a nap or dim light. So, put your blanket and pillows away and sit next to a window.

Typical light boxes, though, come in a wide variety of styles, designs, shapes, colors, sizes, and prices. Savvy shoppers can find good light boxes for well under $200. But you can spend a whole lot more if you're so inclined. And you don't need a prescription to buy a light box.

A variety of professional organizations have endorsed the value of using light boxes for the treatment of SAD. Therefore, some insurance companies may consider reimbursing you for your purchase if your doctor recommends it. Insurance company policies vary widely, and you have to check. If your company refuses, your doctor can help you write a letter of reconsideration. And at the end of the day, if the insurance company refuses, you may be able to obtain reimbursement from a Flexible Spending Account, if you happen to have one available to you at work.

So you have the money, or the insurance coverage, but where do you find the products? Here are places that can get you started:

✔ **www.cet.org:** The Center for Environmental Therapeutics sells bright light and dawn simulation products that have been used in clinical trials.

✔ **www.sltbr.org:** The Society for Light Treatment and Biological Rhythms site has a comprehensive list of manufacturers of light therapy products, which include the e-mail addresses and Web sites of each manufacturer so you can compare and contrast them with each other. Click the "Corporate Members" link.

✔ **www.amazon.com:** This site lists a variety of bright light products along with consumer satisfaction reviews.

Chapter 6

Lightening Up Moods
with Medications

*T*his chapter overviews the various types of medications available for the treatment of seasonal affective disorder (SAD). But before we tell you what you can take, we help you make the decision as to whether you may actually want to pursue this approach. Deciding to take medication for SAD should involve careful consideration of the risks and benefits. The next section takes a look at the good, the bad, and the ugly side of medication.

The most important piece of advice is to collaborate closely with your healthcare professional if you choose to take medication for your SAD.

Weighing the Pros and Cons of Meds

A majority of people can ultimately be treated successfully with medications for their SAD. While not all medications are universally safe, effective, and virtually devoid of bothersome side effects, you can obtain good results through medication if you:

✔ Have a good, collaborative relationship with your healthcare provider

✔ Are willing to take medications

✔ Are willing to experiment with various medications if the first one doesn't help

✔ Are good at remembering to take your medications regularly and as prescribed

✔ Are willing to tolerate at least a few side effects (although these effects often subside and/or can be controlled through additional medications)

✔ Have no contraindications for taking medications (see "Considering the cautions" later in this chapter)

If you're considering medications, check out some of the pluses and minuses in more detail in this section.

Perusing the positives

Taking medication for SAD has certain obvious advantages over other approaches. No doubt, *simplicity* stands first and foremost among these pluses. It's difficult to think of anything much easier and more convenient than taking one or two pills each day. *Speed* is another relatively positive attribute of medications because most antidepressants take between one to four weeks or so to start working.

Cost is a little more complicated. If you have good health insurance, medications for SAD are usually reasonably inexpensive. If you don't have health insurance, you may find that certain medications drain your pocketbook faster than you may think. However, generic drugs can lower costs, and sometimes your physician can offer you samples to help defray a little of the cost.

So, simplicity, speed, and cost are usually considered pros for the medication approach to SAD. Consider medications for a few other reasons:

✔ **You have bipolar disorder or extremely severe depression with psychotic features (see Chapter 2 for types of depression).** Most folks with SAD don't have bipolar disorder. However, if you do, or if your depression is accompanied by seeing or hearing things that aren't there, medications are likely going to be required for successful treatment.

✔ **You feel you have no time for therapy.** In truth, if you feel this way, it may be a symptom of your depression and stress, both of which can be helped with therapy. However, if you think you don't have time for therapy, you probably won't follow through. Therefore, medication may be the thing to try first. After you improve a little, therapy may be an option to consider.

✔ **Light therapy doesn't work or is impossible.** Some people don't respond to light therapy or don't get totally better. Others have eye problems or skin conditions that make light therapy a poor choice. See Chapter 5 for more information about light therapy.

✔ **Your insurance covers medication but refuses to cover light therapy or psychotherapy.** Please realize that insurance companies can sometimes be persuaded to cover psychotherapy or light therapy if you enlist the help of your doctor or mental health professional. However, if your company fails to respond to your request, you may want to try medications.

✔ **Serious suicidal thoughts feel uncontrollable.** When suicide starts feeling like a good option, you need to get help in a hurry. Medications often work a little faster than psychotherapy, which can be important at times like this. However, light therapy can also work very quickly. But whatever approach you take, be sure it's done in close consultation with a mental health professional. You're ill-advised to attempt "going it alone" if you have suicidal thoughts. Fortunately, suicidal thoughts aren't typically a major feature of SAD.

✔ **Your healthcare provider has strong reasons for recommending medications.** Most folks with SAD don't absolutely require medications because other treatment options are at least as effective. However, on some occasions your physician may feel that medications are the way to go for you. If you aren't sure about the recommendation, you can always seek a second opinion.

There may even be times when medication is the best solution, if even only temporarily. Your circumstances at home or your schedule at work may have changed, rendering your normal non-medicine treatments ineffective or even impractical for a time. For example, take a look at Josh's story:

> **Josh** was diagnosed with SAD last year and used light therapy successfully for his treatment. He placed a light box on his desk at work because he needed almost an hour of exposure daily to decrease his symptoms.
>
> This fall, as team manager for a software development firm, Josh is regularly spending 50 hours a week at work. He loves his job and the project. But as time goes on, he loses enthusiasm. He feels exhausted, irritable, and craves junk food. He realizes that he may be having a relapse of SAD.
>
> So, Josh gets out his light box and turns the lights on while working at his desk. However, this year, lights don't seem to be brightening up his mood. He checks with his doctor who asks how much time he spends under the lights. Josh tells his doctor that he's rarely at his desk lately due to the nature of the project he's working on. His doctor asks if Josh has the time to use the lights at home. Josh replies that the next few months mean that he barely has time to read the newspaper in the morning, let alone sit under lights.
>
> Josh's doctor then talks to Josh about considering medication. They agree that, for this year, medication may be an appropriate way to help Josh through the winter season. Medication is a good choice for Josh because he currently doesn't have time to deal with light therapy or psychotherapy. In a subsequent year, he may wish to pursue one of those other options.

Josh is proactive in dealing with his SAD. He recognizes what's happening early on and promptly seeks help from his doctor when his normal course of treatment (light therapy) doesn't do the trick. He's a good candidate for medication because the options of light therapy and psychotherapy are too time consuming this year. After his project is complete or the seasons shift to warmer weather, there's a good chance Josh can come off the medication.

Considering the cautions

Although antidepressant medications are quite convenient and have been shown to work effectively for all types of depression as well as SAD, sometimes you may not want to take this route. Some medications have various disadvantages, downsides, and contraindications.

A *contraindication* is when there are factors present making what would normally be a safe solution risky. For example, if you're a woman, a medication that's usually safe may not be safe if you become pregnant. Or, because certain medications don't play well together, you need to avoid taking two medications that are contraindicated with each other.

Other cautions include the following:

- ✔ **Cost:** If you read the section earlier in the chapter about the advantages of medications, you may think we're a little coo-coo. But cost can be a disadvantage too, especially when you don't have good health insurance. If you're forced to pay out of pocket, medicines can get pricey. A relatively small number of people with SAD may need to take medications for as long as six months or more out of every year. Over many years, the cost of even modest co-pays, mounts up.

- ✔ **Distressing side effects:** Side effects of most antidepressant medications lessen somewhat if you stick it out for a while. Other times, healthcare providers can add another medication to help control the side effects or switch you to something else that won't cause so much trouble. But some people simply find almost any side effect irritating. And sometimes the side effects can be pretty severe, and each new medication seems to involve new complications. Such side effects can include weight gain, nausea, dry mouth, sexual dysfunction, and headaches.

- ✔ **Discontinuing difficulties:** Although antidepressant medications aren't considered to be addictive in the usual sense, some people do experience significant distress during the tapering off period. A few experience flu-like symptoms, increased anxiety, and a variety of other physical complaints. Usually, these symptoms are mild and manageable as long as you work carefully with your doctor on a withdrawal plan.

✔ **Pregnancy and/or breastfeeding:** This issue is a little controversial. A few experts contend that at least some antidepressant medications are quite safe, even for breastfeeding or pregnant women. And if you happen to be seriously suicidal, whatever risks that do exist are probably overridden by the seriousness of your symptoms.

But most folks with SAD aren't highly suicidal, and insufficient data exists to conclude that these medications are absolutely safe for pregnant/breastfeeding women. For example, recent evidence has suggested that certain antidepressant medications (SSRIs, see "Checking Out Medication Options for SAD" later in this chapter) may cause a slight increase in risk for heart-related problems in the infant when the mother takes the drug during pregnancy. And babies may even have some difficulty in withdrawal from medications when their mothers have taken them while pregnant. For most people, too many other good treatment options exist to recommend antidepressants for SAD.

✔ **Personal philosophy:** Some people have a strong personal preference for avoiding medications. In the case of SAD, that's okay because various other, effective treatment options exist (all are reviewed throughout this book). However, if nothing else works for you and your mental health professional advises it, we hope you reconsider.

✔ **Suicide risk:** There has been concern about an increase in thoughts about suicide in children, adolescents, and young adults taking antidepressants of various types. This concern may apply to older adults as well, although we simply don't know for sure at this time. The U.S. Food and Drug Administration recommends that people taking antidepressants see a doctor once a week for the first month and three more times in the next two months. Yet, a recent study found that most children and adults don't see a mental health professional in the first month after beginning an antidepressant.

Adverse drug events are a leading cause of accidental death throughout the world. These events occur when people mix medications with other medications, over-the-counter (OTC) medications, alcohol, or other substances. Most of the time these deadly mixes are unintentional and, if not deadly, result in emergency room visits, hospitalizations, and sometimes permanent damage. That's why it's so important to be open and honest with your healthcare providers about all the medications, vitamins, alcohol, and drugs that you use or take. Especially mention any herbs or supplements you take because they can interact with medications. Even an occasional drink, when mixed with certain medications can result in an adverse drug event.

Heather's story illustrates the concerns about taking medications when considering becoming pregnant.

Heather, the mother of a rambunctious 2-year-old son, is constantly delighted by her child. She enjoys taking him for walks in his stroller and sitting at the park talking to other moms in the neighborhood. October is filled with sunny and warm days. The winds bring in the first snow on Halloween night. Winter arrives suddenly, and November turns dark and frigid. Rain, snow, and sleet mix with cloudy days. Heather finds herself wishing for the return of long walks and visits to the park but knows that spring lies a long way off.

Her son seems to be more demanding and difficult to amuse. Heather loses patience with him. She resents getting up early with him. She feels overcome by constant fatigue and falls into bed, napping when he does. She's considered having another baby but now wonders if she's a good enough mother and if she can handle the additional responsibility.

During a regular visit to her nurse practitioner, Heather breaks down in tears. After taking a careful history, the nurse practitioner brings up the possibility that Heather may have SAD. She talks about the treatment options and the good news that SAD (and other forms of depression) can be successfully treated. Heather is hopeful and believes that she may have been suffering from SAD during previous winters. However, after considering the options, she and her healthcare provider decide that medication may not be appropriate because Heather wants to become pregnant. Heather is referred for brief cognitive-behavioral therapy (see Chapters 9 and 10).

Neither Heather, nor her nurse practitioner want to run any risk while she's considering becoming pregnant. Although most antidepressants aren't known to cause serious problems with a developing fetus, there haven't been enough studies on this issue to conclude that no risks exist for the baby. Cognitive-behavioral therapy represents an excellent choice for someone in that position.

Heather's story shows that there are various treatment options for people with SAD. When there are reasons to avoid medication, hopeful possibilities remain.

Understanding How Antidepressants Work

Overall, antidepressant medications represent a success story for the pharmaceutical industry and a lifesaving remedy for millions of people who have benefited from them. These medications target the chemical messengers in your brain known as neurotransmitters.

The first antidepressants were found by a serendipitous stroke of luck. Doctors treating tuberculosis in the 1950s noticed that their patients taking the drug *Iproniazid* demonstrated a surprising surge in their spirits. From there, researchers explored other formulations for treating depression.

Billions of nerve cells called *neurons* comprise the brain. Neurons process information that comes in from both inside the body and the outside world. Neurons communicate by sending chemical messengers called neurotransmitters across the gap that lies between them. These neurotransmitters appear to be disrupted by mood disorders such as SAD. Scientists have discovered more than 300 different types of neurotransmitters. However, most antidepressant medications appear to primarily affect

- ✔ **Dopamine:** Dopamine disruptions are related to problems with attention, arousal, motivation, and addiction.

- ✔ **Norepinephrine:** Problems with Norepinephrine appear to cause difficulty with lethargy, decreased energy, and reduced mental alertness.

- ✔ **Serotonin:** This neurotransmitter affects memory, mood, sleep, and anxiety and seems especially involved in SAD and other types of depression.

Medications sometimes affect only one neurotransmitter whereas others affect two or more. Furthermore, they affect these neurotransmitters in different ways. Some drugs boost certain neurotransmitter levels; other medications block the reabsorption of neurotransmitters thereby increasing their levels; still others do things that are more technical than you want to know about. Many antidepressants are identified by which neurotransmitters they effect. The most common class of antidepressants increase serotonin and are known as selective serotonin reuptake inhibitors (SSRI's). Check out the section "Checking Out Medication Options for SAD" later in this chapter.

Today, you have dozens of medication choices for the alleviation of SAD. But most research on antidepressants has been conducted with people suffering from a major depressive disorder (see Chapter 2) and not specifically from SAD. Nevertheless, because SAD involves depression, most researchers believe that the majority of antidepressants work fairly well for SAD.

But, the puzzle of what specific drug helps a particular person presents quite a conundrum to psychiatrists and other professionals who prescribe these medications. Some people respond quickly to the first medication they take and experience almost no side effects. Others experience severe side effects and sometimes must try a half dozen or more possibilities before they experience any relief. However, the answer to this problem may lie just around the corner (see the sidebar "The promise of pharmacogenetics").

More help is on the way

Hormones are another type of chemical in the body that affect moods. Melatonin (a hormone) levels may be disrupted in people with SAD (see Chapter 3 for info on melatonin). In addition, cortisol (a hormone released when you're stressed) may be disturbed in about half of the folks with depression. The nature of the disturbance seems to involve the cycle or rhythm of cortisol secretion. People with depression usually have abnormally high levels of cortisol all day, and the levels don't decrease in the evening and at night. Excessive levels of cortisol have also been related to high blood pressure and heart disease. Researchers are hot on the trail for producing medications that target problems with various hormones and neurotransmitters associated with mood disturbances.

If you start taking an antidepressant, you should be followed closely by a mental health professional, especially in the first couple months of treatment. Without treatment, depression can be disabling and deadly. Experts believe that although medication may occasionally and temporarily increase suicidal thoughts, the benefits of treatment outweigh the risks. In fact, medications actually appear to reduce suicidal risks over the long term.

Checking Out Medication Options for SAD

The good news about SAD is that there are a variety of medication options. The bad news is that there are a variety of medication options. In other words, you may find the array of possibilities a little confusing. Don't fear. The following information is broken down to the essentials. Read it and discuss your concerns and questions with your doctor.

Medications typically have official scientific names and a variety of trade names that sometimes vary a little according to subtle differences in formulation. For example, "SR" after a drug name usually means "sustained release," and "XL" designates "extra long." The basic ingredients are essentially the same in these variations, but the duration of action may vary somewhat.

Wellbutrin

Bupropion (most commonly known by its trade name, Wellbutrin) is the first antidepressant medication that has been *specifically* approved by the Food and Drug Administration (FDA) for the treatment of SAD. A number of studies have now been carried out and have demonstrated that Wellbutrin appears to be effective in the treatment of SAD as compared to placebos.

The selection of Wellbutrin for treating SAD wasn't entirely random. There are many potential benefits:

- Researchers felt that Wellbutrin would be especially effective for SAD because it doesn't usually cause sedation or weight gain. Because fatigue and weight gain typically accompany SAD, doctors figured that a medication that didn't worsen those symptoms would be a good idea.

- Wellbutrin doesn't typically cause sexual dysfunction like many other antidepressants do.

- Wellbutrin can be prescribed in the early fall before symptoms begin and discontinued in the spring when symptoms generally improve. Prescribing Wellbutrin in this manner, in effect, means that this medication can actually prevent the symptoms of SAD from reoccurring.

- Wellbutrin is also used to help you quit smoking (prescribed under the trade name of Zyban).

- Wellbutrin has been found to be useful for some people with attention deficit disorder (aka ADD or ADHD).

- Wellbutrin boosts the available levels of norepinephrine and dopamine in your brain. These neurotransmitters are associated with energy, alertness, attention, and motivation.

However, Wellbutrin doesn't prevent SAD symptoms for everyone, and some people report little or no benefit from Wellbutrin. Side effects, the part you always hear mumbled rapidly in television drug commercials, can be significant. Such side effects can include:

- Anxiety
- Constipation
- Dry mouth
- Extreme anxiousness or agitation
- Hypertension
- Insomnia
- Mania (see Chapter 2)
- Nausea
- Shakiness
- Sweating
- Weight loss

The promise of pharmacogenetics

The first antidepressant prescribed to an individual patient may work quite effectively. Unfortunately, in over a third of the cases, relief from depression either doesn't occur or the side effects are very distressing. That's why many people give up on antidepressants before they find one that works for them. And that's a shame because a large majority of people ultimately find a medication that works well — when they and their doctors persist in the search. The new science of pharmacogenetics helps identify the genetic factors that predict who's most likely to benefit from what medication. Pharmacogenetics may also help identify who's likely to experience problematic side effects from any particular medication.

Psychiatrists and specialists at the Mayo Clinic developed a blood test (cytochrome P450) that provides information about a specific patient's probable response to an antidepressant. This area of research is new and exciting. Researchers believe that the next few years of study will allow more precise prescribing of antidepressants. Even more importantly they expect that this research will lead to the development of new classes of antidepressant medication specifically tailored to an individual's genetic profile. That's why you want to tell your doctor about any close family member who's experienced success with antidepressant medication. There may be a genetic reason to consider that same medication for you.

If you have a history of seizures or are at risk for seizures, provide your doctors with this information because Wellbutrin, especially at high dosages, can occasionally trigger seizures. Doctors generally steer patients away from Wellbutrin if they

- ✔ Have had a recent head injury
- ✔ Have had an eating disorder
- ✔ Are withdrawing from alcohol or sedatives
- ✔ Have nervous system tumors
- ✔ Are pregnant or breastfeeding
- ✔ Have a history of bipolar disorder (see Chapter 2)
- ✔ Are taking certain other types of antidepressants
- ✔ Are allergic to Wellbutrin

Obviously, Wellbutrin should be prescribed by a healthcare provider who's very familiar with this specific medication. The provider should meet with you regularly, at least for the first few months. Side effects can often be managed successfully. Be sure to report any difficulties you experience.

Selective serotonin reuptake inhibitors (SSRIs)

Selective serotonin reuptake inhibitors (SSRIs) basically increase the availability of the neurotransmitter serotonin in the brain (see the section "Understanding How Antidepressants Work" for more information). They're the most widely prescribed antidepressant medications. Since Prozac, which came to market in the '80s, these drugs have replaced most of the older forms of antidepressant medication because the side effects, while substantial for some people, are much less severe than those medications that preceded SSRIs. More importantly, an overdose of an SSRI is almost never deadly.

Prozac and Zoloft

Two SSRIs that work for the treatment of SAD are Prozac and Zoloft. Both have been found to be more effective than taking a sugar pill (placebo) in treating SAD.

- ✔ **Prozac:** Prozac is also known by the generic name of *fluoxetine* and is a reasonable choice for people with SAD. Prozac works by increasing the availability of serotonin (as well as boosting norepinephrine and dopamine neurotransmission). Prozac can improve mood and decrease anxiety. It's prescribed for SAD, major depression, certain anxiety disorders, some eating disorders, and premenstrual disorders.

- ✔ **Zoloft:** This drug, known generically as *sertraline,* is also an SSRI that usually boosts energy. Like Prozac, it increases the amount of serotonin in the brain. Zoloft is prescribed for SAD, depression, and anxiety. In addition, Zoloft likely increases dopamine neurotransmission.

Taking Prozac or Zoloft often results in an immediate boost in energy. This side effect makes sense for SAD sufferers many of whom sleep too much and report chronic feelings of fatigue. However, improving mood usually takes more than a week or even up to 4 weeks. If you don't get relief in a month, talk to your doctor. You may need an increase in your dose or another medication.

So, what are the downsides to taking an SSRI? Well, one that's particularly bothersome for some is the common side effect of sexual dysfunction. This can mean lack of interest or even delay or lack of orgasm. If this is a problem, other medications can be tried or added. Don't suffer in silence. Talk to your doctor.

Most side effects from taking Prozac or Zoloft go away over time. So, if you aren't too uncomfortable, the best plan is to wait a few weeks. But some side effects are so unpleasant that they can't be ignored or tolerated. Here are a few:

- ✔ Agitation
- ✔ Apathy or emotional flattening
- ✔ Diarrhea
- ✔ Insomnia
- ✔ Loss of appetite
- ✔ Nausea
- ✔ Sweating
- ✔ Weight loss

If you suffer from side effects, don't abruptly discontinue your medication. SSRIs may need to be tapered off. Talk to your doctor to see if there are other ways to manage the side effects, and if you decide to stop taking the medication, do so with your doctor's help.

Other SSRIs with potential for SAD

There's every reason to think that the other SSRIs may be effective for the treatment of SAD. Studies for this application simply haven't been carried out, but they've been shown to effectively treat other types of depression. Side effects vary a little from drug to drug but tend to be similar to the ones from Prozac and Zoloft (discussed in the preceding section). Don't be surprised if your healthcare provider prescribes one of these medications (especially if Wellbutrin, Zoloft, or Prozac didn't work for you):

- ✔ **Celexa (Citalopram):** This medication doesn't work quite as quickly as its cousin, Lexapro (next bullet). But it has been found to be particularly well tolerated by the elderly. Celexa is also known for its relatively mild side effects.

- ✔ **Lexapro (Escitalopram):** This drug works a little faster than other SSRIs. It can be taken safely with many other medications. Lexapro tends to have milder side effects than the other SSRIs.

- ✔ **Luvox (Fluvoxamine):** This SSRI may be used if you suffer from insomnia because it tends to be sedating. You probably won't be prescribed Luvox if you have the more typical SAD reaction of oversleeping. This drug is often used for people with anxiety. Luvox has a few more gastrointestinal side effects than many of the SSRIs.

✔ **Paxil (Paroxetine):** This SSRI is also used frequently for people who have both depression and anxiety. This medication tends to be a little sedating, so it wouldn't be a usual first choice if you tend to oversleep or have fatigue. Paxil has been associated with weight gain in some people. Stopping Paxil can be more difficult than going off other SSRIs so be sure to talk with your doctor before you make that decision.

More medication choices for SAD

Some antidepressant medications affect different neurotransmitters in different ways than the SSRIs. Although research showing them to be effective for the treatment of SAD is sadly lacking, they may ultimately prove to be effective for SAD. Some of these medication options include the following:

✔ **Cymbalta (Duloxetine):** Cymbalta is one of the newer antidepressant medications on the market. It's prescribed for depression and has been approved by the FDA for the treatment of chronic pain associated with diabetes. This drug acts by increasing serotonin, norepinephrine, and dopamine. Cymbalta is often prescribed for lack of energy or for chronic aches and pains.

✔ **Desyrel (Trazodone):** This medication affects serotonin in different ways than the SSRIs. Desyrel is often prescribed for insomnia — so if your SAD symptoms include sleeping too much, this drug may not be for you. Desyrel is sometimes prescribed as a medication to be taken with other medications that cause insomnia.

✔ **Effexor (Venlafaxine):** This medication increases serotonin, norepinephrine, and dopamine. Effexor works a little faster than many antidepressants and has relatively few adverse drug interactions. It may work when one of the SSRIs hasn't done the trick. Unfortunately, Effexor is usually contraindicated for people who have cardiovascular disease or high blood pressure.

✔ **Norebox or Edronax (Reboxetine):** This drug increases norepinephrine and dopamine in the front part of the brain. It can cause insomnia and agitation. This energizing medication can be helpful for people with fatigue and lack of motivation, and it doesn't cause weight gain. For those reasons, this drug may be a good candidate for the more common symptoms of oversleeping, weight gain, and lack of energy. Norebox is widely available in many countries, but not in the United States.

✔ **Remeron (Mirtazapine):** This drug is a good choice for people with insomnia. The drug increases both serotonin and norepinephrine. Remeron is usually sedating and has been associated with weight gain, so this drug may not be the one for you if you suffer from those problems. On the plus side, Remeron may cause fewer sexual side effects.

Considering Golden Oldies

The older antidepressant medications haven't completely faded away with the development of the newer medications. The newer antidepressants discussed in the preceding sections in this chapter typically have fewer side effects and are less lethal when overdosed. Yet, prescribers still turn to the older medications when a particular person doesn't respond to a newer antidepressant. Professionals may also consider the older medications to augment or boost the effectiveness of another antidepressant. These older antidepressants consist of two major categories: Tricyclics and MAO inhibitors.

Tricyclic antidepressant (TCA) medications

Tricyclic antidepressant (TCA) medications increase the levels of serotonin and norepinephrine and to a lesser degree, dopamine. They were the most popular antidepressants during the 1960s and into the 1980s when the SSRIs were discovered (see "Selective serotonin reuptake inhibitors [SSRIs]" earlier in this chapter).

TCAs typically have more side effects than the newer drugs, so you should probably not consider TCAs if you have

- Cardiac problems
- Diabetes
- Enlarged prostate
- Glaucoma

On the other hand, TCAs do work fairly well for depression. Interestingly, they've also been used to treat chronic pain (such as migraine headaches, fibromyalgia, and back pain), bedwetting in children, and some eating disorders. A few tricyclic medications that are widely prescribed include

- **Anafranil (Clomipramine):** This TCA is prescribed for depression, pain, and obsessive-compulsive disorder (OCD). Anafranil is somewhat sedating, so if fatigue is part of your SAD, you may want to steer clear.

- **Asendin (Amoxapine):** This medication has been used for depression that's accompanied by anxiety or agitation. Weight gain and sedation are common side effects. The drug shouldn't generally be used by the very old or young or people with Parkinson's disease.

> ✔ **Elavil (Amitriptyline):** This TCA is also used when people experience pain with their depression. Again, weight gain and sedation are common. It's good for insomnia and so-called treatment-resistant depression. However, its tendency to cause sedation and weight gain can rule it out for many people with typical symptoms of SAD.

Other tricyclic medications include

✔ Ludiomil (maprotiline)

✔ Norpramin or Pertofrane (desipramine)

✔ Pamelor or Aventyl (nortriptyline)

✔ Sinequan (Doxepin)

✔ Surmontil (trimipramine)

✔ Tofranil (imipramine)

✔ Vivactil (Protriptyline)

If you're prescribed a tricyclic medication, be sure to ask your doctor about the choice. You want information about effectiveness and side effects.

MAO inhibitor medications

MAO inhibitor antidepressant medications work by blocking the enzyme monoamine oxidase, which destroys other neurotransmitters such as serotonin, norepinephrine, and dopamine. So if less of those neurotransmitters are being destroyed, you have a larger quantity available in your brain. And these medications work pretty fast.

MAO inhibitors are occasionally prescribed for resistant depressions and treatments or depressions with unusual features. The MAO inhibitors include

✔ Emsam (selegiline) — see the sidebar "A possible resurgence for MAO inhibitors?"

✔ Nardil (phenelzine)

✔ Parnate (tranylcypromine)

✔ QMarplan (isocarboxazid)

Unfortunately, MAO inhibitors also come with side effects and warnings:

✔ They can be responsible for elevations in blood pressure because they cause a build up of something called tyramine.

✔ If you're taking an MAO inhibitor, you must avoid cheese, alcohol, fish, meat, avocados, sausage, yogurt, caffeine, and chocolate.

✔ They're contraindicated for almost any cardiac problem.

✔ MAO inhibitors are usually only prescribed when other medications have failed.

✔ Because of potential dangerous side effects and interactions with other drugs, MAO inhibitors should only be prescribed by an expert in psychopharmacology.

Looking Beyond Typical Antidepressants

Sometimes your healthcare provider may turn to a type of medication that isn't classically considered an antidepressant. Two types of these "non-antidepressants" exist that you should know about — mood stabilizers and atypical antipsychotics.

Sometimes these medications are lifesavers. However, they can have some very serious complications. Make sure that you have a collaborative relationship with your prescriber — you want to know what and why you're being prescribed one of these and if there are safer alternatives.

Mood stabilizers

Mood stabilizers were originally developed to treat either seizures or manic episodes that go along with bipolar disorder (see Chapter 2). They're sometimes used to supplement the treatment of depression by combining them with other antidepressant medications.

Side effects of mood stabilizers vary but can include weight gain, interference with birth control, tremors, rash, and overdose. Make sure you keep in close contact with your doctor if you take a mood stabilizer.

Lithium

Lithium is the most common mood stabilizer, and it's been around for a long time. Lithium can be added in small doses to other medications to enhance treatment. Side effects such as tremor or delirium (disorientation and confusion) may indicate a dangerous toxic reaction.

A possible resurgence for MAO inhibitors?

Due to concerns about dangerous food and drug interactions, MAO inhibitors have largely fallen into disfavor. However, new versions of these medications hold out greater promise. One in particular comes in the form of a transdermal patch called Transdermal Selegiline. It has been approved as part of the treatment for Parkinson's patients and major depressive disorders. Transdermal Selegiline has been used in clinical trials and found to be safe and effective for depression. More research is needed, and it has yet to be studied in the treatment of SAD.

Other mood stabilizers

The other common mood stabilizers are often used to treat seizures. However, they're sometimes given in addition to other antidepressants in order to stabilize moods. These medications include

- ✔ Depakote (valproate)
- ✔ Lamictal (lamotrigine)
- ✔ Neurontin (gabapentin)
- ✔ Tegretol (carbamazepine)
- ✔ Topamax (topiramate)

Some of the mood stabilizers have shown intriguing potential to treat a few disorders other than depression. These applications include Topamax for alcoholism, gambling, and migraines; Neurontin for chronic pain, Tegretol for nerve pain, and Lamictal for nerve pain.

Atypical antipsychotics

If you're depressed and your doctor prescribes an atypical antipsychotic, you may be shocked. The term *psychotic* refers to a person who's lost contact with reality and may experience delusions, paranoia, and hallucinations, none of which have probably occurred with you if you have SAD. But these drugs have the potential to aid in treatment of non-psychotic depressions, which is often an off-label use. Your doctor may consider them when other treatments haven't been as successful.

Atypical antipsychotics are also known to have mood-stabilizing effects, meaning they calm you down and lessen mood swings from high to low. The side effects of the antipsychotics can be very serious. But the good news is that most SAD sufferers don't require these drugs. Nevertheless, side effects can include

✔ Heart rhythm disturbances

✔ Hypotension (low blood pressure)

✔ Problems with regulating temperature

✔ Seizures

✔ Tremors

✔ Weight gain (sometimes substantial)

Common atypical antipsychotics include the following:

✔ Abilify (aripiprazole)

✔ Clozaril (clozapine)

✔ Geodon (ziprasidone)

✔ Invega (paliperidone)

✔ Risperdal (risperidone)

✔ Seroquel (quetiapine)

✔ Solian (amisulpride) (not available in the U.S.)

✔ Zyprexa (olanzapine)

Chapter 7

A Happy Diet for SAD

*I*n this chapter, you discover the connection between seasonal affective disorder (SAD) and food. We offer tips on healthy eating, which may also improve your mood a little. But getting yourself to eat healthy isn't always an easy thing to do, especially if you're depressed. So you also get ideas on changing both your behaviors and your eating environment in ways that improve your chances of maintaining healthier eating habits.

Substance abuse is also a big issue with SAD. You read about the common problem of substance abuse and ways to avoid that trap. The chapter rounds out with ways of using your thinking to keep you on the right path.

The Mood/Food Connection

People suffering from SAD or the winter blues often experience increased appetite or food cravings. Typically those cravings focus on foods that produce a rapid rise in blood sugar levels. These foods include simple carbohydrates, such as candy, soda, chips, and doughnuts. A rise in blood sugar gives you a quick boost in energy and for that matter a boost in your moods.

The problem is that these same foods absorb quickly, and the boost in mood and energy is short lived. Therefore, the craving quickly returns because the blood sugar drops rapidly and the body demands more. It's sort of like trying to keep warm by continually feeding your fireplace with newspapers instead of logs.

Complex carbohydrates, on the other hand, burn slowly. Foods like whole grains, vegetables, beans, and fruits (not fruit juice) absorb more slowly into the body. And they produce a longer, steadier burn so cravings don't return as quickly.

For many SAD sufferers, allowing moods and cravings to drive what and how much they eat ultimately leads to undesired weight gain.

In fact, Dr. Raymond Lam, an expert on SAD at the University of British Columbia, reported that 10 percent of his SAD patients gained more than 20 pounds during the winter season. Sadly, when people put on unwanted pounds, they often feel guilty, ashamed, have lower self-esteem, and increased depression. These negative feelings then lead to more cravings to temporarily boost moods. And the beat goes on.

Breaking the cycle and putting your eating habits on more healthy footing improves your overall well being. Healthy habits help lift your mood and allow you to better manage your SAD.

Regaining and keeping control of your eating uses four tactics: motivation, monitoring, managing, and menu planning. People who attempt to change their eating patterns find that motivation is a struggle. They start out with great intentions and then find themselves going off course. The next section gives you tips on maintaining your focus on eating right.

Motivating Your Mind

More often than not, SAD leads to overeating and extra pounds. When it does, you may want to diet and lose weight, but you just don't have the willpower. Actually, thoughts like "I don't have enough willpower" just don't help. In fact, those kinds of thoughts sabotage the best of intentions. Such negative thinking is another common symptom of SAD (see Chapter 9 for more information about SAD and your thoughts). SAD can drain your enthusiasm and motivation like pulling out the plug of a bathtub full of water.

The truth is that you can use your mind to increase your motivation or to defeat yourself before you even get out of the starting blocks. To get motivated, try calculating costs and benefits and making new associations.

See Chapter 15 for even more information about how to motivate your mind. The techniques described for getting yourself to exercise can also be applied to developing new ways of eating.

Carbs and melatonin

Melatonin is a hormone secreted at night by the pineal gland in the brain. Melatonin causes drowsiness and a drop in body temperature. People with SAD appear to have higher levels of melatonin during the daytime in the winter than people who don't experience SAD. Intriguingly, carbohydrates do the opposite — they increase energy and body temperature. Researchers speculate that the reason people with SAD may crave carbohydrates is to counteract the effects of their excessive melatonin levels. Bright light treatment (see Chapter 5) appears to reduce melatonin levels in people with SAD. And some researchers have speculated that light therapy may prove to be useful in helping folks with SAD regulate their weight and carbohydrate cravings.

For more information about melatonin, see Chapter 3.

Calculating costs and benefits

So where do you find your fountain of willpower? In your head — and through a cost/benefit analysis of changing your eating patterns. A cost/benefit analysis is essentially a way of tallying the advantages and disadvantages of making changes of almost any kind, including new ways of eating healthy. The reason that using this tool is helpful is because people often are unaware of the reasons that making a change can truly benefit or in some cases, cost them. Writing out these costs and benefits clarifies the issues and helps sustain the motivation needed for lasting change. Using Anthony's story and the steps to follow, you can complete a cost/benefit analysis for your eating habits:

> **Anthony** looks forward to his retirement. He's worked for 35 years and put away enough to live very comfortably. One of his plans is to sell his house in Minnesota and move to Florida because his SAD has plagued him much of his life.
>
> But at 6'4" and 280 pounds, he fears that he could die of a heart attack before enjoying much of this phase of life. He's already taking medications for his blood pressure and cholesterol. His doctor tells him that he must increase his exercise and lose weight. Anthony loves pizzas, ice cream, and junk food. He struggles with finding the motivation to make a sustained effort at changing his eating. So he fills out a cost/benefit analysis for changing his eating in order to discover whether making changes in his eating feels worth the effort it takes.

Table 7-1 shows you Anthony's Cost/Benefit Analysis Form. You can find a blank copy in Appendix A. Here are the steps to creating your own analysis:

1. **Use Table 7-1 to diagram your analysis.**

2. **At the top of the form, write your goal (you can also use this strategy for a decision or a problematic thought — see Chapter 10 for applying this approach to thoughts).**

   Your goal doesn't have to be about changing your eating; that was Anthony's goal though.

3. **In the left-hand column, write about all the conceivable costs of making the changes you want to make.**

   Put down your deepest fears and concerns.

4. **In the right-hand column, write down all of the imaginable benefits that your goal could bring you, and make sure to be creative.**

5. **Under your chart, make a section called *My Reflections.***

   Record what your cost/benefit analysis taught you. In this section, include your thoughts about minimizing the costs.

Table 7-1	Anthony's Cost/Benefit Analysis
Goal: Changing to healthy eating.	
Costs	**Benefits**
I'll feel deprived. I hate that.	I'll live longer.
I'll feel hungry all the time.	I'll be healthier.
I won't be able to enjoy meals out with my friends. What kind of life is that?	Maybe I can even get off some of my medications; I don't like the side effects.
I can't watch TV without munching on snacks.	I'll have more energy.
I love the taste of potato chips, and I'd miss that.	I won't get teased so much about my weight.
I couldn't celebrate good times without feeling a loss.	It'll be easier to exercise, which I used to enjoy.
	I'll feel better about myself.
	I won't have to ask for a seatbelt extender on airplane trips.

Costs	Benefits
	I'll worry less about dropping dead from a heart attack; sometimes I even have panic attacks over that issue.

My reflections: This situation is a no-brainer. Clearly the payoff is worth it. I actually don't have to feel all that deprived if I go slow and do it right; they say that deprivation isn't the way to accomplish healthy eating. I can eat healthy and still enjoy TV, my friends, and so on. I can substitute frozen yogurt for ice cream, and I can eat rice cakes (some of which are really tasty) that can work instead of potato chips. Overall, I'll feel better and have better health. I'm going to do this!

Anthony discovered that he has more than enough reasons to undertake a lasting change in his eating patterns. He also realizes that some of his perceived costs of changing aren't as bad as he originally thought. He wants to enjoy his well-earned retirement in good health. The cost/benefit analysis helped him see all of these issues more clearly than he had.

Making new associations

Another way to motivate your mind is by creating new, positive associations between what you do and what you eat. As it stands right now, you probably have certain celebratory foods linked in your mind to many happy events. For example, cake and ice cream with birthdays; chips and chicken wings to watching sports; champagne with promotions, and so on.

SAD suffers associate winter with various problematic eating styles. Thus, hot chocolate goes hand in hand with cold winter nights. And you may even associate heavy stews, breads, and other comfort foods with staying warm in the winter. However, these associations are simply due to habit, and they can be changed.

Start a few new associations for your mind. Try linking healthier alternative foods to special occasions. For example, look up recipes for lower calorie desserts and snacks. Serve fresh fruit with low-calorie, low-fat dips. Sparkling water with a lime slice can substitute for soda. Even baked chips, though not perfect, are healthier than fried. Warm alternatives for the winter include hot tea, healthy low-fat soups, and low-fat lattes.

Watch out for enemy number one: trans fatty acids. See section below on Fighting fats for more information about trans fatty acids and their dangers.

Monitoring Food and Triggers

Research indicates that anything you can do to increase your *awareness* helps you make changes in your behavior. When you run on autopilot, you may be unaware of what you're doing and resort to old habits.

Monitor and track your food and what triggers your food cravings. Keep a food diary to make you aware of what you've been eating. People who write down what they eat tend to lose weight. Tracking your food triggers includes listing the times, situations, or moods that lead to food cravings and snacking.

Ava's story shows how monitoring her moods and food cravings helps her maintain focus on healthy eating:

> **Ava** uses light therapy in the fall and winter to help her control her SAD. She still craves carbs in the winter, but her moods are generally better. At her yearly physical she's surprised when her doctor tells her that her blood tests indicate that she's at risk for getting diabetes. She's only about 15 pounds over her ideal weight and hadn't been too concerned about it, but her doctor explains that she carries her extra weight all in her abdomen, increasing her risk. He wants her to make some changes in the way she eats. He also tells her that stress can lead to weight gain. Her doctor suggests that she use a food diary to track her moods, foods, and triggers for her eating. He explains that keeping such records can help her develop alternatives to eating at critical, high-risk times.

Table 7-2 shows you Ava's Food and Trigger Diary. You can find a blank copy of the Food and Trigger Diary in Appendix A. Here are the steps to creating your own diary:

1. **Diagram a table like Table 7-2.**

   Every time you eat or you're tempted to eat, write down the day and time.

2. **In column two, write down what was happening at the time of your temptation.**

   If it is simply a mealtime and nothing else was going on, just record *breakfast, lunch,* or *dinner.*

3. **Jot down your mood and what you were feeling at the time of eating in column three (see Chapter 9 for more information about feeling words).**

4. **In column four, record everything you ate and approximately what quantity (serving size or calories).**

   If you craved food, but didn't eat it, write that down too.

5. At the end of each day, write a *My Reflections* response.

Write a few sentences about your observations. Try not to be harshly judgmental, but record what you've discovered about your eating habits from that day's diary entries.

Table 7-2	Ava's Food and Trigger Diary		
Day/Time	*Event*	*Mood*	*Food or Craving*
M/7:00 a.m.	Breakfast; late for work	Rushed, anxious	Grabbed a muffin and then at work I wolfed down two donuts
M/10:15 a.m.	Team meeting	Bored	Two bagels and had a big glass of juice
M/12:30 p.m.	Lunch	Sad	Hamburger and super-sized fries
M/7:30 p.m.	Dinner	Tired and cranky	A large frozen pizza and a soda
M/8:30 p.m.	Watching TV	Stressed and tired	Two bowls of Rocky Road ice cream

My Reflections:

Well, I'm going to try not to beat myself up here. But I can sure see where my moods link to my mindless eating. One thing I need to do is go to the grocery store and buy healthier food to have around. Things like frozen pizzas are just too easy to fix. I also see that I need to bring some healthy food to work instead of eating all those bagels and donuts they have at work. I also see I'm too stressed and unhappy at work; maybe I can ask for more help. My doctor said too much stress leads to weight gain around the abdomen. I can see where keeping track of my eating is going to start changing my behavior.

Ava found that keeping track of her food cravings, moods, and triggering events helped her see problematic patterns in her eating. She was turning to food to deal with stress and low moods. This awareness enabled her to come up with alternative strategies at key, high-risk times.

By being aware of your food triggers, you can choose to substitute other behaviors for eating. Substitutes include

- ✔ **Drinking hot green tea:** Instead of indulging in soda, drink green tea, which contains antioxidants and increases your metabolism.

- ✔ **Drinking ice water:** Drinking water is good for you, and it helps fill your stomach, easing hunger pangs. Cold water may even give your metabolism a small kick as well.

✔ **Going outside:** Instead of reaching for that leftover drumstick, get up and step outside. Doing so is good for your SAD because of the light and good for your mood. While you're at it, take a short walk.

✔ **Breathing:** Step away from the chips, and take five minutes to do some slow, deep breathing. See Chapter 11 for more details on using breathing to deal with moods and difficult emotions.

✔ **Reading a good book:** Reading can distract you from food cravings and even activates more brain cells than watching television. Pick up a book and put down the candy bar! And don't read cookbooks . . .

✔ **Slowing down:** Most experts also recommend that you consume your meals slowly. The body takes about 20 minutes to signal the brain that you're full. The only problem with that is that studies also show that most folks eat a whole lot faster than that. Therefore, it's not a bad idea to actually time how long it takes you to eat for a while. Try to stretch it out by chewing longer and pausing between bites.

✔ **Monitoring your weight:** About once a week, at the same time of the day, weigh yourself and record the result. Numerous studies show that people who regularly weigh themselves don't gain as much and have more success at their efforts to lose weight. If you weigh more often, be sure not to take the day-to-day fluctuations too seriously. Various factors influence how much water weight you have on any given day.

Over concern about calories and weight can be a red flag that you could have an eating disorder. Remember, balance is the key. Eating disorders involve excessive dieting, bingeing, and sometimes purging. If you have any signs of these problems, seek professional assistance and stop weighing yourself in the meantime.

Managing Food Intake

Everyone wants quick, easy solutions to their problems. Yet, most problems don't come with easy buttons. That's why they're problems. Change takes effort. The same goes for eating. A healthy diet requires managing your food intake.

SAD sufferers typically crave carbohydrates, load up on high-calorie foods, and don't pay attention to what or how they eat. Treating SAD through light therapy, behavior therapy, or cognitive therapy can actually reduce some food cravings. But it's a good idea to focus on the food part of the problem as well. Healthy eating starts with reducing calories and also includes ways of managing your style of eating.

Reducing calories

You can't get around calories. Take in more than you need; you gain weight. Consume less than you need; you lose weight. Most people know that. But what they don't know is that about 3,500 calories results in about 1 pound (and 1,575 calories equals about one kilogram) of weight. That means that if you take in 100 calories per day less than you need to maintain your weight, you inevitably lose about 10 pounds in a year and 30 pounds in three years.

Exactly what does it take to cut out 100 calories per day? It's a lot easier than you may think. Here are some very simple ways:

✔ Drop the cheese from one hamburger

✔ Drink a glass of water instead of juice

✔ Go from regular mayonnaise to fat-free mayo or yogurt

✔ Drink fat-free milk rather than whole milk

✔ Use fat-free salad dressing

✔ Cut out one glass of wine or a beer

Alternatively (although it's better to do both), you can easily exercise 100 calories off per day. You don't even have to join a gym. Here are a few easy ways to do that each day:

✔ Walk quickly around the house or around the block for 15 minutes.

✔ Ride a bike for 10 minutes.

✔ Get a pedometer and monitor how many steps you take the first day, and then add an extra 2,000 steps (to your first day's steps) each day.

✔ Swim for 15 minutes — do laps or tread water.

Do you make bad food choices when you come home late and want to fix something quick and easy? To overcome that obstacle, prepare a number of meals in advance on the weekend and freeze serving sized portions that are quick to reheat in the microwave. In many cities, personal chefs perform this service, and you can visit places that help you prepare a week's worth of delicious, healthy food in advance.

Seeing your food

When you eat, most of the time, you have no clue about how much you've eaten. And yet most people *think* they're pretty good judges of what they've eaten. The truth is that what your eyes tell you has a lot more to do with how you judge your consumption than what your stomach has to say.

Double your loss?

You can double your weight loss by cutting out 200 calories per day through decreased food consumption and/or exercise. But don't cut out more than around 250 calories per day because when you attempt to lose more than about a half pound per week, your body attempts to sustain its weight by slowing your metabolism. Thus, you have a much harder time accomplishing your goal. But guess what? Most dieters try to lose more than that amount and therefore end up in a self-defeating battle of loss of and regaining weight.

If you want to succeed at dieting, go slowly and avoid making yourself feel terribly deprived or even extremely hungry. Strong feelings of deprivation and/or hunger lead to overeating. Go slow and steady. The pounds won't slough off as quickly, but they remain off. The number-one reason most people fail at dieting is that they try to lose weight too fast.

Dr. Brian Wansink (Director of the Cornell University Food and Brand Lab) and his colleagues have conducted numerous experiments on the issue of food and perception. One of our favorites was a clever experiment in which they rigged soup bowls to partially refill as diners were eating their soup. Thus, the people had no visual cue to tell them how much they'd consumed. Person after person consumed far more soup than people who ate out of regular, non-refilling soup bowls. Diners with the refilling bowls ate almost twice as much soup as the others, but reported that they'd eaten about the same amount as people eating from normal soup bowls. The lesson from this and similar research is that your eyes tell your brain more about what you've eaten than does your stomach. Counterintuitive, to be sure, but true.

So, how do you make use of this information? Here are several useful suggestions:

- **Put everything on your plate that you plan to eat.** For example, don't eat your snacks out of boxes or large bags because your eyes have no cues for knowing how much you've eaten.

- **Use small plates and small glasses.** This idea may sound a little silly, but 3 ounces of cottage cheese on a small plate looks like a lot more food than 3 ounces on a large dinner plate.

- **Avoid distractions.** When you're watching television, reading a book, even talking with other people, your eyes don't notice what you've been eating. People eat much more food when they're distracted. Try to make your eating the primary focus whenever you can.

- **Anticipate distractions.** When you do have distractions coming up such as parties and restaurant meals, plan ahead and think carefully about what you order and try to at least focus some of your attention on what you've consumed.

Pushing it back

People automatically, without thinking, reach for foods that are immediately accessible. (We used to put candy out in our waiting room. Unfortunately, we ended up eating more of it than our clients did. It was just too tempting. Now our waiting room just has magazines.) People with SAD often have trouble concentrating so they may be at higher risk for eating reflexively without conscious awareness of what they're doing.

Anything you do to make food less convenient and a little more burdensome to get to makes a huge difference. You may even find yourself thinking about food less and eating less. Here are a few ways you can make food less automatic and less convenient:

- ✔ **Put the tempting stuff in back.** Take the rich deserts and other goodies and put them in the back of the refrigerator or cupboard. Make them a pain to reach. Have some carrots, celery, and such at the front.

- ✔ **Stash the leftovers.** After you cook your food, serve it up and put the leftovers away. You can still go back and get more if you really want to, but you may just do it less often.

- ✔ **Don't buy junk food in the first place.** Keeping ice cream, cookies, or candy around is a path to disaster. When you do purchase them, buy in small quantities so you can't eat as much, even if it costs a little more that way.

- ✔ **At restaurants, box up first.** When you order a meal at a restaurant, realize that most establishments serve too much! Ask your wait person for a box when you make your order instead of after your meal. When your food comes, box up half of the meal right away.

Making a Better Menu

The winter is such a hassle for folks with SAD so most sufferers do little to plan their menus. They turn to quick frozen entrees, fast food, and stuff that comes right out of the box. As they eat this way, weight increases. Then they feel badly about themselves. Those bad feelings lead to more eating.

If you're eating the wrong stuff, we have some suggestions. Yes, it involves a little bit of effort. However, the payoff of healthy eating can be substantial.

Going back to nature

The body's digestive system was designed to break down unprocessed foods. In the olden days of horse and buggies, sugared cereals or French fries on the go didn't exist, and people were rarely overweight. Today, food processing factories take the place of the body's digestive system and serve up food that's absorbed too rapidly (even though it may taste great and quickly boost energy and moods). Most dieticians believe that this increase in processing has contributed to the obesity epidemic in the modern world.

Therefore, you should seek unprocessed foods whenever you can. These foods come in the form of fruits, vegetables, and whole grains. Also make sure to keep your consumption of processed foods to a minimum — toss out the white bread and switch to whole grain. When you can, look for the words "stone ground 100 percent whole wheat." Eating foods made with white flour is almost as bad as eating sugar. If you want to be even more scientific about your search for foods that digest slowly, consider taking a look at what's known as the glycemic index.

Think of the glycemic index as an odometer for your food. The glycemic index tells you the speed at which food is digested and converted to glucose by the body. In other words, it rates foods based on their net effect on blood sugar levels. The general rule of thumb is that the slower that speed, the less effect on blood sugar levels. That's because longer digestion helps maintain blood sugar at relatively more constant levels with fewer peaks and valleys. Food that digests rapidly has a high (fast) glycemic rating. For example, a doughnut has a glycemic rating of about 76, an apple has a rating of 36, and kidney beans 27. If you struggle with carbohydrate cravings (whether you have SAD or not), choose foods with a low glycemic rating. These ratings are available in various books and on the Internet. In general, the lower the rating, the slower the absorption, and the better for you.

Fighting fat

Diet plans used to condemn almost all fat. Then for a while, some diets told you to eat nothing but fat and protein. Most nutritionists today don't advocate either of those approaches. Fat doesn't necessarily make you fat. But your body needs a certain amount of fat to sustain healthy organs and efficient brain function. Furthermore, this fact may surprise you, but a small amount of fat can actually slow the absorption of sugars.

The kind of fat you consume makes a big difference:

✔ **Hydrogenated oils or trans fats:** The worst fats go back to the issue of processing. Hydrogenated oils or trans fatty acids have been processed into a goo that clogs your arteries and raises your risk for heart disease. It's so bad for you that a growing number of cities either have or are considering banning trans fatty acids from restaurants. If you see the words *partially hydrogenated* or *hydrogenated* on a food label, that food has trans fatty acids. These fats are found in abundance in cookies, chips, crackers, and many other processed foods.

Eat your oatmeal the right way

Oatmeal is often touted for its health benefits. Labels boast of oatmeal's cholesterol-lowering effects. But the type of oatmeal you eat may make a big difference. Steel cut oats are whole grains that are coarsely chopped. Their glycemic rating is about 42. It's worth looking for steel cut oats on the shelves because instant or quick cooking oats have a glycemic rating of 82. That's because the additional processing makes them cook faster and more importantly, digest quicker.

You may think the 30-minute cooking time sounds like a pain, but you can always make a large batch of steel cut oatmeal on Sunday morning and put the extra into a large plastic container and refrigerate it. Then you can heat up small servings throughout the week in the microwave. Put a little fresh or dried fruit on top, and the oatmeal makes a healthy, delicious breakfast. If you pour milk on top of your oatmeal, don't forget to use low-fat or nonfat milk.

✔ **Monosaturated fats:** Monosaturated fats are beneficial when consumed in moderation. These fats are contained in nuts, olives, and seeds. Monosaturated fats may also confer some health benefits by decreasing the harmful effects of cholesterol. They may have important antioxidants as well.

Olive oil, a monosaturated fat, makes a healthy alternative to butter for bread or sautéing vegetables.

✔ **Polyunsaturated fats:** Polyunsaturated fats don't cause as much harm as saturated fats (see the next bullet). Vegetable oils such as sunflower and corn oil are polyunsaturated fats. They remain liquid at room temperature. Unlike their cousins (saturated fats), these fats in limited quantities may actually protect you from health problems.

Omega-3 is an especially important polyunsaturated fat, contained in fish, flax seed, and some other grains and nuts. See Chapter 8 for more information about special uses of Omega-3 oils in the possible treatment of SAD.

✔ **Saturated fats:** Saturated fats aren't good for you. They include animal fats within meat, coconut oil, and palm oil, as well as the fats contained in butter and cheese. Saturated fats raise your bad cholesterol (LDL) and increase your risk of heart disease.

Avoid trans fats (first bullet point) and saturated fats as much as you can. You don't have to give up entirely on meat and cheese, but limiting intake is wise. Focus on healthy fats and consume them in moderation.

If you mostly consume so-called healthy fats, you should attempt to limit your total fat intake. That's because fats contain about 9 calories per gram as compared to 4 calories per gram in carbohydrates and protein. Therefore, an ounce of fat contains more than twice as many calories as an ounce of carbs or protein. So would you rather fill up on a tablespoon of butter or 200 grapes? The calories are the same.

Rationing out your protein

A number of fad diets have suggested consuming mostly protein while others have minimized its use. Protein is essential for repairing and building new cells. Protein supplies amino acids that are necessary for the manufacture of the body's neurotransmitters that control moods. Protein also helps you feel full and satisfied.

What you need to know about protein is pretty simple:

- ✔ Have a little protein at every meal.
- ✔ Eat low-fat protein when you can — that means skinless chicken breasts are better for you than fried chicken.
- ✔ Low-fat yogurt is a good source and better than ice cream (well, a better choice that is).
- ✔ Probably the best and healthiest source of protein are beans because they're low fat and high in fiber.

Putting fiber in your diet

Most folks don't get enough fiber. There are two types of fiber, and they're both good for you:

- ✔ **Insoluble fiber** binds to water, which creates bulk and makes you feel full. It keeps your digestive system going to help produce bowel movements. Whole grains, wheat breads, and vegetables contain insoluble fiber.
- ✔ **Soluble fiber** is broken down by bacteria and binds to fat in the intestines and lowers cholesterol. You find soluble fiber in oatmeal, citrus fruits, and beans.

How much fiber should you eat? There's no absolute answer to that question, but it appears that most people consume less than half the fiber that they should. Recommendations typically range from about 25 grams of fiber per day up to 50 grams. People over 50, especially need fiber to maintain health.

The Pitfalls of Alcohol

People with SAD are very susceptible to cravings for sweets and other carbohydrates. More seriously, they can also be at risk for abusing alcohol. This abuse happens for a number of reasons. SAD sufferers already struggle with painful, difficult feelings. They feel anxious or have trouble falling asleep. It's very tempting to turn to alcohol to feel better, relax, or to help fall asleep.

The problem is that alcohol is obviously addictive, and it can make the quality of sleep worse (that is, reduced REM or dream states). Furthermore, alcohol has a whole lot of calories. Just two glasses of wine each day can add up to 20 pounds of extra weight in a year! In addition, mixing alcohol with medications can be a very bad idea.

On the other hand, many studies have shown that a low consumption of alcohol may confer health benefits. Up to two drinks per day for men and one drink per day for women may have cardiovascular benefits.

Before you start "drinking for your health," check with your doctor and discuss any risk that you may have for abusing alcohol. It isn't worth starting to drink for the health benefits if you have any such risk. And if you currently suffer from SAD, you may be at some risk of abusing alcohol.

So how can you determine if you have a drinking problem? Because SAD can impact your reasoning, there's a way to at least make an initial assessment. Just answer the CAGE questionnaire! Be brutally honest in each of your answers:

- ✔ **C:** Have you ever felt you needed to **Cut** down on your drinking?

- ✔ **A:** Have people **Annoyed** you by criticizing your drinking?

- ✔ **G:** Have you ever felt **Guilty** about drinking?

- ✔ **E:** Have you ever felt you needed a drink early in the morning (**Eye-opener**)?

The more of these questions you answer with *yes,* the more concern you should have. A *yes* to even one of these questions is cause for some concern. If *any* of the above bullets apply to you, get some more information. A great resource is www.behaviortherapy.com. The site has a terrific, research-based drinkers' checkup that can offer more insight into whether alcohol is a problem for you.

If you think you may be experiencing a problem with alcohol, get help. You can also try reading *Addiction & Recovery For Dummies* by Brian F. Shaw, PhD, Paul Ritvo, PhD, Jane Irvine, D. Phil, and M. David Lewis (Wiley), which provides you with a lot of useful information. See Appendix B for more resources for substance abuse problems.

Chapter 8

Alternative Treatments for SAD

· ·

· ·

*I*n the 1860s, during construction of the Transcontinental Railway, Chinese workers shared their snake oil with others as a remedy for joint pain. Apparently, the Chinese claimed that oil from Chinese water snakes contained an anti-inflammatory agent (and there may have been some truth to it). However, unsavory salesmen substituted inert ingredients for the snake oil, promoted its use as a remedy for nearly everything (not just joint pain), and flooded the market with phony promises and shady sales gimmicks. The term "snake oil salesman" is now associated with dubious claims for miracle cures as well as unethical business practices.

Unfortunately, in this age of science, snake oil salesmen still exist. Infomercials proclaim the benefits of special treatments, and the media reports on the latest fads promising simple solutions to complex problems. Lose weight, live healthy, get rich, be happy. People with seasonal affective disorder (SAD), like anyone else with a problem, can easily become seduced by offers of a quick or easy fix.

In this chapter, you discover how to evaluate the sources of treatments so you won't fall prey to false claims. Then you take a look at alternative remedies for depression and SAD.

Alternative remedies are a range of treatments that currently aren't considered primary, frontline approaches to treating SAD. For each of these treatments, we let you know what research has shown — for better or for worse. Please consult with your medical doctor or therapist before you try unknown or unproven remedies.

Evaluating the Data

Almost daily there seems to be another report on some new medication, treatment, diet, or lifestyle change that increases longevity, decreases pain, improves mood, or cures illness. The newspapers, the Internet, magazines, books, and television all tout the latest remedies, all claiming to be the most effective. Obviously, you can't believe everything.

When you hear about new treatments for SAD (and you *will* hear about them), how can you sort out the truth of legitimate studies from sloppy science and downright fraudulent advertising? The task may seem daunting, but you can get a better idea about the validity of a new claim by considering the source and taking a closer look.

Checking the reliability of the source

So, you just read an article about a new "cure" for everything from SAD to toenail infections. If the cover of the periodical you're reading includes sensationalistic headlines about alien kidnappings, celebrity escapades, or losing 50 pounds in less than a month, run the other way! Tabloids and the like may be entertaining, but they rarely contain useful information on new medical treatments.

But just because you're reading a more serious magazine, doesn't guarantee the information is solid either. Look for information about the credentials of the authors of a particular study. The authors (those folks who conducted the research) should've earned degrees, such as a PhD, MD, RN, MSW, PharmD, or MS. The research should be sponsored by a university, medical school, government agency, or reputable research institute. If the sponsoring agency sounds at all questionable, you can check it out through your library or with other professionals in the field.

Be cautious about where you get your information. Genuine research studies are reviewed by experts when published in scientific journals. Good magazine articles or news reports identify where the original research was conducted and published.

Even authors with good credentials sometimes have financial ties to the research they report. For example, a pharmaceutical company may be footing the bill for the research. Although you may not always know about those ties, good journals require authors to report them. And sometimes the financial ties are obvious, such as when an expert appears in an infomercial.

Looking more closely at actual studies

When buying a car, whether you're a mechanic or not, odds are you look under the hood. Do the same with medical research. Most of you probably aren't experts or even want to be experts at analyzing research. However, you need to watch out for a few issues when looking at reports on new treatments:

- ✔ **Make sure that any new treatment has shown good results *more than a few times.*** Never trust a single study or two. Science works by an accumulation of knowledge and replication over time.

  Be a little skeptical of studies involving just a few people. Such studies are suggestive at best. You can't rely on testimonials or a couple of case examples. Generally, treatments don't become fully accepted until many studies have found consistently positive results in randomized controlled trials.

- ✔ **Check to see if a report on a new treatment states whether the findings came from a study that included random assignment to various experimental and control groups (aka, a *randomized controlled study*).** If the study involves drugs, it should also be conducted on a double-blind basis. That means that neither the researchers nor the participants know who's getting the "real" drugs versus a "placebo (a pill with no real effect, popularly referred to as a sugar pill)."

- ✔ **Talk with your healthcare provider.** Your primary care provider (PCP) is likely to know something about most alternative treatment methods. Keep your provider informed about alternative treatments you've tried, are currently using, or are considering. Doctors and nurses today are reasonably supportive of alternative treatments that have shown some degree of effectiveness.

Assessing Alternative Approaches

A very large percentage of people turn to alternative treatments for both depression and SAD. Alternative remedies are a range of treatments that currently aren't considered first approaches to treating SAD. Many alternative treatments are safe and reasonably compatible with standard treatments, but some can pose problems such as drug interactions, allergic reactions, or other undesirable side effects.

You can sit back and relax and read this section. We've done the scientific analysis for you on some alternate treatments for SAD. We take a look at three groups of alternative treatments:

- ✔ **Internal:** These treatments are over-the-counter (OTC) supplements or other treatments that you swallow or breathe in.

- ✔ **External:** Therapies that involve external touch.

> ✔ **Radical treatments:** These much-less-common medical therapies are provided by doctors when mainstream treatments have failed to work.

All accepted treatments start out as alternatives until research has repeatedly verified their effectiveness. So don't get discouraged from considering alternatives. In many cases, they're worth a try, at least as a complement to standard therapies for SAD. If you happen to have an unusually resistant form of SAD, keep searching. New, promising treatments are always under development.

Internal alternatives

Internal alternatives include nutritional supplements that can be obtained without a prescription in grocery stores, drug stores, and health food stores. Negative ions are another "internal" alternative that involve changing the electrical charge of the air you breathe. The quality and number of studies backing these approaches vary quite a bit.

Increasing your melatonin

Melatonin is a naturally occurring hormone produced by the pineal gland located just above the middle part of your brain. The pineal gland receives information concerning when to produce melatonin from the body's clock, technically known as the suprachiasmatic nucleus (SCN) within the hypothalamus gland (see Chapter 3). And in turn, the SCN receives its information from the eyes. Light signals the SCN, which signals the pineal gland to stop producing melatonin.

By contrast, darkness turns on the flow of melatonin. Melatonin has been referred to as the Dracula hormone. That's because, like Dracula, melatonin comes out at night, in the dark.

Because winter days are shorter and dark periods last longer, you may assume that melatonin levels would generally be higher for people in the winter months. In fact, that's true for folks who suffer from SAD. Interestingly, people who don't fall prey to SAD maintain constant levels of melatonin across the seasons (see Chapter 3 for more information on why that may be the case).

So if SAD sufferers have more melatonin in the winter months, the last thing you want to do is suggest that they take more melatonin, right? Well, actually melatonin can possibly benefit you by helping to regulate your circadian rhythms.

Researchers at the Oregon Health and Science University randomly assigned people with SAD into three groups. The first group took melatonin in the morning and a placebo in the afternoon. The second group took a placebo in the morning and melatonin in the afternoon. The third group was given a placebo to take in both the morning and the afternoon. For most of the sufferers, receiving melatonin in the afternoon (as compared to placebo), decreased their depressive symptoms.

Although melatonin may have a variety of possible uses, including the treatment of SAD, be aware of the number of cautions:

- ✔ Melatonin is considered a food supplement in the United States, and its manufacture isn't regulated by the government; therefore, the actual doses you receive may vary from manufacturer to manufacturer.

- ✔ Some people have strong reactions to melatonin, including drowsiness, dizziness, nightmares, headaches, or nausea.

- ✔ Don't take melatonin if you're pregnant or breastfeeding; enough info isn't out on how it might affect your baby.

- ✔ Don't take melatonin before you drive or operate machinery (because of the drowsiness factor).

- ✔ Realize that the number of studies supporting the effectiveness of melatonin for SAD are somewhat limited at this time.

- ✔ If you do decide to take melatonin for SAD, consult your physician, psychiatrist, or a sleep specialist because the timing and dosing are different for everyone.

- ✔ You may see melatonin touted for the treatment of a wide variety of other ailments including cancer, heart disease, infertility, and even for extending longevity. Research to date, while fascinating, is far from the point where melatonin's effectiveness can be established for these applications at this time.

Melatonin has been found to be useful for some people who experience jet lag, too. A variety of studies support this use for melatonin. Generally, taking it within an hour or two of bedtime at the arrival destination is useful. Melatonin may also help with insomnia, especially for people who have trouble with sleep onset.

Using St. John's Wort

St. John's Wort, a weed that grows wild in meadows, has anti-inflammatory and antibacterial properties and has been used medicinally to treat a wide variety of ailments in people. Today, St. John's Wort is primarily being used to treat depression — mild to moderate cases. Although results have varied somewhat, St. John's Wort appears to be about as effective as many prescription antidepressant medications and may have even fewer side effects.

But this seemingly miracle-type supplement does present some downsides for SAD sufferers:

✔ Because SAD is a type of depression, St. John's Wort may seem like an ideal treatment, but one of the side effects is photosensitivity (sensitivity to light), which can result in sunburns or eye damage from sunlight. Because one of the primary treatments for SAD is bright light therapy (see Chapter 5) as well as increased exposure to the sun in general, St. John's Wort may not be a good choice for treating most cases of SAD.

✔ St. John's Wort is known to produce negative interactions with various prescription medications. Consult your doctor and/or pharmacist.

✔ St. John's Wort is considered a supplement, and manufacturers don't have to adhere to the same quality standards as pharmaceutical companies. Therefore, dosages may vary, and contaminates sometimes appear in some formulations.

Consult with your PCP if you're considering treating your SAD or other type of depression with St. John's Wort. In the case of SAD, do *not* combine it with bright light therapy.

Ingesting omega-3: The "fishy" alternative

The body of evidence indicating the value of omega-3 in the treatment of depression is relatively small but highly suggestive. Interestingly, omega-3 oils were first found to have value in adjunctive treatment of cardiovascular problems. For example, it has been found to reduce triglyceride levels, decrease blood pressure, and reduce the risk of fatal heart attacks. But some cynics of omega-3 believe that not enough research exists on the use of omega-3 because omega-3 can't be patented, and drug companies can't make any money on it.

Nevertheless, the research that does exist on omega-3 and depression is pretty good. Some trials have shown that omega-3 works. The exact recommended dosage isn't yet well established, but two grams per day is commonly well tolerated and apparently effective. Taking omega-3 if you have depression makes pretty good sense but again as a complement to other more established treatments.

You can get your daily does of omega-3 fatty acids from cod liver oil, cold water fish (such as salmon), flaxseed, avocados, and more conveniently, in supplements. Taking fish oil helps decrease depression.

If you're pregnant or breastfeeding, be careful about eating fish known to have a high mercury content (and sometimes other contaminants) such as shark, sword fish, mackerel, tile fish, and tuna. Some people even have rare cases of allergic reactions to fish and some nuts that contain omega-3; people with diabetes should consult their doctor prior to supplemental consumption of omega-3 because diabetes is a complex disorder with various medications required, which could interact with omega-3. Furthermore, internal bleeding can occur from very high doses of omega-3.

Positively fighting your mood with negative ions

Negative ions are odorless, tasteless, and invisible particles that you inhale in certain environments such as around beaches, waterfalls, following thunderstorms, and even in your shower at home. Some researchers have suggested that negative ions may boost production of serotonin and might have benefits for depression and SAD (see Chapter 6 for information about the role of serotonin and SAD).

A few good randomized controlled studies of treatment with negative ion generators have demonstrated improvements in SAD that were superior to placebo and equivalent to light therapy. Participants typically have been exposed to the generators for about 30 minutes per day for good results.

You can buy negative ion generators at high-end gadget retailers or from the Internet. But buyer beware — it's difficult for the ordinary person to know if the ionizer truly produces a good flow of negative ions. One study conducted at Columbia University showed that different machines varied greatly in their output.

Not only is it difficult to know the quality of the generator you might buy, but also studies remain few in number. And most of the research has been carried out at a single laboratory. Scientists like to see replication at various labs before uniformly endorsing new therapies. On the other hand, there probably isn't much harm or risk associated with negative ion therapy.

Taking supplements

A variety of supplements for the treatment of depression have been proposed. And if they work for depression, they probably work for SAD:

- ✔ **5-HTP:** This supplement is a building block for serotonin. Increasing serotonin levels has been associated with improvements in depression. The jury is out on whether this supplement works efficiently to improve SAD.

- ✔ **SAM-e:** This supplement is used in Europe for the treatment of depression, and a few studies have shown SAM-e to be more effective than a placebo. However, these studies are few in number and not of uniformly high quality. Furthermore, SAM-e costs more than most supplements.

- ✔ **Vitamin D:** A number of investigators have speculated that vitamin D may be helpful in improving SAD. Exposure to the sun increases vitamin D production in the body, so one randomized, controlled study found that vitamin D decreased SAD symptoms. However, the study was quite small and hasn't been replicated.

Most of the above supplements aren't regulated in the United States, and they've received little research attention to date. Therefore, we can't recommend them to you at this time. Talk to your doctor for recommendations.

External alternatives

External treatments involve your sense of touch. We discuss two general external strategies (acupuncture and massage). There are variations on each of these approaches (for example, acupressure, Reiki massage, and so on), but scientific research is lacking on the relative effectiveness for these variations.

Getting the point of acupuncture

Practitioners of Chinese medicine have utilized acupuncture for thousands of years. Acupuncture involves inserting extremely fine needles into specific sites of the body in order to balance a theorized flow of energy through the body. In Chinese medicine, all illness is considered to emanate from imbalances in energy flow. Such energy is called *qi* or *chi* (pronounced *chee*).

After the needles are in place, they're manipulated, heated, and/or run a very slight electric current through them. Western medicine believes that acupuncture works by causing a release of endorphins. Endorphins are substances, produced by the body, similar to opium, that elevate moods.

This procedure may sound painful, but it isn't usually. Acupuncture has received increasing acceptance in Western medicine in the past couple of decades and has been used to treat a surprisingly wide array of disorders including headaches, back problems, nausea from chemotherapy, fibromyalgia, and tennis elbow.

Only a few studies have looked at acupuncture for the treatment of depression. Results were positive, but the data to date is insufficient to recommend this approach as a primary treatment for SAD. The good news is that acupuncture is quite safe when performed by a licensed, well-trained professional. Ultimately acupuncture may prove to be reasonably effective for SAD. In the meantime, there probably isn't any harm in trying acupuncture as a complement to other, better-established treatments for SAD.

Massaging away SAD

Dim lights, quiet music, pleasant aromas, oils, and warm, positive attention often form a backdrop to massage therapy. And most people find that massage — the rubbing or manipulation of the body's soft tissues — is both pleasing and relaxing. Massage appears to increase positive moods, decrease anxiety, lower blood pressure, slow the heart rate, relieve aches and pains, and promote a sense of well being.

Massage doesn't appear to have been studied in the specific treatment of SAD. However, because it has shown positive results for general depression, it does seem likely that massage could benefit people with SAD. Therefore, we enthusiastically recommend obtaining as many massage therapy sessions as you can realistically afford if you have SAD. Or you might convince your partner (if he or she is willing) to administer massage. Basically, any type of massage that feels good and doesn't hurt you is likely to improve your mood — at least temporarily. (Here's the rub: Almost all the studies conducted to date for the treatment of depression with massage have only looked at depression levels at the end of a series of treatments. Therefore, we simply don't know whether the effects endure. Common sense suggests that the effects may be fleeting.)

Massage therapy can have a few downsides. For example, unless you have a very nice and willing partner, it can get rather expensive over time. And be careful if you have cancer (avoid massaging the area of a tumor), burns, open wounds, or a serious injury of any type. If massage hurts — don't do it.

For the time being, consider massage largely as a complement to the better-established treatments such as cognitive therapy (see Chapters (9 and 10), behavioral therapy (see Chapters 14 and 16), medication (see Chapter 6), or bright light therapy (see Chapter 5).

Radically Treating Resistant Depression

Generally speaking, SAD is quite treatable. Most sufferers can expect a good outcome from conventional approaches that may or may not be comple-mented by one of the strategies noted in this chapter. However, a small minority of folks with SAD may have or develop a type of depression known as treatment-resistant depression. *Treatment-resistant depression* fails to remit even after a number of different treatments have been tried.

The strategies in the following sections have been used primarily only for severe, treatment resistant depressions. They shouldn't be considered with-out medical consultation and aren't for the faint of heart — and all of these treatments involve the use of electricity in different ways.

Vagus nerve stimulation

Vagus nerve stimulation was originally developed for treating epilepsy that didn't respond adequately to medication. Some of these epilepsy patients reported improvements in mood following treatment. No one knows for cer-tain how this approach works on depression, but the research backing the effectiveness of vagus nerve stimulation is very preliminary and highly con-troversial. However, here's what's involved.

First, a surgeon implants an electrical pulse generator into your chest. Then a wire is run from the gadget and attached to your vagus nerve, which communi-cates between your brain and other major organs of your body. The generator sends electrical impulses to your vagus nerve at regular intervals. Although a few patients have reported benefits, the jury is far from reaching a verdict.

Side effects of this therapy can include changes in voice, hoarseness, cough, difficulty swallowing, some breathing difficulty when exercising, and neck pain. If the battery wears out in the generator, you need more surgery to replace it.

Using magnetic fields

Two kinds of treatment for depression involve magnetic fields:

- **Transcranial magnetic stimulation (TMS):** This treatment uses electricity to generate a powerful magnetic field, but doesn't apply electricity directly to the body or brain. A paddle with a wire coil transmits a magnetic field to the brain. A few small studies have shown TMS to decrease symptoms, but the evidence is scant at this time.

- **Magnetic seizure therapy (MST):** In this case, the fields trigger a controlled seizure in the brain. We don't know why, but this therapy usually produces rapid relief from treatment resistant depression.

Doctors hope, but don't yet know for sure, that both types of magnetic stimulation will result in less cognitive impairment and memory loss than electroconvulsive therapy (ECT) — described in the next section. Be aware that the research for both of these treatments is very preliminary. In fact, one study found that TMS worked no better than a "sham" or "placebo" treatment.

Getting shocked out of depression

Electroconvulsive therapy (ECT) isn't used as a first approach to the treatment of depression and is generally limited to severe, resistant cases. The main concern with ECT is that it can cause cognitive impairments and memory loss. And the memory losses can build up and persist with repeated administrations.

This approach to treatment-resistant depression sounds the scariest of all to most people. ECT evokes images of old horror movies. The truth is a little more serene. Today, ECT takes place under controlled conditions. The patient is sedated, and electrodes attach to one or both sides of the brain. Electricity is used to trigger a controlled seizure.

Part III
Shifting SAD Thoughts

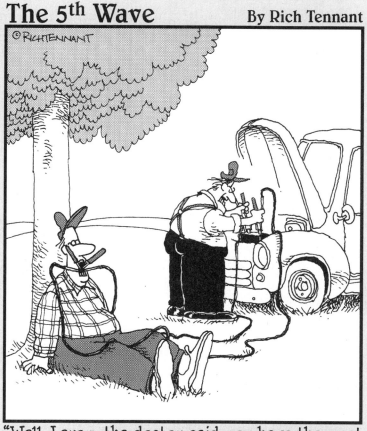

The 5th Wave   By Rich Tennant

"Well, Leroy, the doctor said you have the most treatment resistant SAD he's ever seen and suggested electric shock therapy. I sure hope he knows what he's talking about."

In this part . . .

Cognitive therapy is a well-established, research based, approach for the treatment of depression and numerous other disorders. Recent research has shown that cognitive therapy works just as well for seasonal affective disorder (SAD) as it does for other emotional problems. In this part of the book, we help you identify problematic SAD thinking and give you ways of improving your thoughts.

We also provide you with tools for managing the emotional storms that come with SAD, and finally we provide some tips for decreasing the stress in your life.

Chapter 9

Exposing SAD Thinking

*P*eople suffering from seasonal affective disorder (SAD) typically internalize negative and pessimistic beliefs and feel unable to deal with everyday problems. Fortunately, helping folks change the way they think helps them feel better and live their lives more fully. Literally hundreds of studies support the value of thought therapy for the treatment of depression.

For decades, thought therapy (aka cognitive therapy) has been used successfully to treat depression. Thought therapy is based on the principle that the way you interpret or think about yourself, events, and the future affects the way you end up feeling.

To illustrate the relationship between thoughts and feelings, imagine that on a bitter cold, winter day you slip on a patch of ice. Ouch! You think one of three ways:

✔ "I'm an idiot, a total klutz." You feel quite upset with yourself, maybe even embarrassed.

✔ "Some jerk failed to clean off this sidewalk." You feel annoyance or anger at someone else.

✔ "Gosh, I'm glad I didn't break any bones!" You feel a sense of relief that you're unhurt and not heading to the emergency room.

This single event can yield three different emotions, all because of how you choose to think about or interpret the event of slipping on the ice.

In this chapter, we show you how SAD-influenced thoughts can darken and distort your view of winter, yourself, the world, and your future. You get strategies for tracking your thoughts, feelings, and the events that trigger them. People often find that their thoughts and feelings change for the better simply by monitoring them. But if you don't find that to be the case, Chapter 10 gives you a wide selection of strategies for changing your thinking.

Fishing for Feelings

SAD sufferers feel pretty miserable when their SAD is active. Yet, the synonymous terms, *cognitive therapy* and *thought therapy* may lead you to think that feelings aren't an important focus for this type of therapy.

Sure, the most obvious cause of SAD is the body's reaction to reduced sunlight in the winter. This biological response includes disruptions in circadian rhythms, which significantly alter body chemistry (see Chapter 3 for more info). So why would thought therapy have any value in treating SAD?

For a long time no one tried treating SAD with cognitive therapy, at least not in formal studies. Light therapy was seen as the treatment of choice (see Chapter 5). Fortunately, a light bulb went off in psychologist Dr. Kelly J. Rohan's (from the University of Vermont) mind. She thought that cognitive therapy may be very effective in treating SAD. Her notion makes sense because changing the way you think not only changes the way you feel but also changes brain chemistry. Thus, if you figure out how to have thoughts that are less gloomy and more upbeat, the levels of neurotransmitters in your brain will also change for the better. Furthermore, British scientists (Drs. David Healy and J. M. Williams) reviewed research that indicated that improving one's thinking may help restore normal circadian rhythms. So if cognitive therapy can improve brain chemistry and normalize circadian rhythms, thought therapy can brighten up the moods of SAD sufferers.

Research by Dr. Rohan and her colleagues confirms that cognitive therapy is very effective in the treatment of SAD. Initial studies suggest that thought therapy works *at least as well as* light therapy for SAD and may actually be better at preventing relapse in the future.

The whole point of thought therapy is to help you feel better. But first, you have to recognize what you're feeling. Feelings are words or concepts that describe your emotional state. In essence, these words provide a label for a variety of bodily sensations that occur in response to events. In order to truly know what you're feeling, you need to become aware of your bodily sensations and then connect feeling words to those sensations. Don't worry if you don't get it yet; the examples in this chapter can guide you.

For example, you may notice your heart racing, your breathing becoming rapid and shallow, and your hands trembling. If you pay attention to these bodily sensations, you may be able to realize that the feeling word related to them is *fear*. In someone else, the same bodily sensations may connect to the feeling word, *angry*. And others may not be able to describe the feeling associated with those sensations at all.

In fact, many people are truly out of touch with their feelings. They distance themselves from their true feelings in a variety of ways. Denial, taking it out on others, and falling apart all represent ways that people avoid facing their true feelings. Not being aware of your feelings makes change much more difficult. Think about the way you handle your feelings. Do you ever find yourself using one of these ways of distancing yourself from your feelings:

- **Choosing denial:** Do you convince yourself that everything is just fine even when it isn't? For example, one SAD sufferer kept telling us, "I'm perfectly okay." But his wife clearly saw that he was lethargic, sleeping poorly, and eating more junk food than usual.

- **Taking it out on others:** Do you redirect your misery onto other people or even the dog? For example, a person with SAD may become easily irritated over just about anything while blaming others for everything that goes wrong. That person may also deny feeling depressed while friends and family can see clear signs of a depressed mood.

- **Falling apart:** Do you act in immature or helpless ways? People with SAD may act overwhelmed when facing minor stress. They ask for help when it isn't needed and neglect their usual responsibilities such as bill paying, grocery shopping, and cleaning. They appear depressed to people who know them but remain unaware of their true feelings.

Casting a line to catch feelings

Do you think you may be out of touch with your feelings? Do you sometimes feel out of sorts but are unable to put your feelings into words? If that describes you, it's time to reconnect with your feelings.

Here's a step-by-step exercise that can help you get a better handle on your feelings:

1. **Pull out a notebook that you can carry around easily for a day or two and create what we call a Fishing for Feelings Chart.**

   Draw lines to create three equal columns on the first few pages.

2. **Label column one, *Bodily sensations,* column two, *Feelings,* and column three, *Event.***

3. **Set aside four or five times each day to spend a minute or two noticing your bodily sensations.**

   Write them down in column one. The types of sensations to notice include the ones listed below (as well as anything else you may notice about your body's reactions):

   • Cold or shivering when environment is temperate

   • Diarrhea

   • Dizziness

   • Fatigue

   • Goosebumps

   • Headaches

   • Heaviness in chest

   • Hot and red in a cool setting

   • Increased or decreased appetite

   • Increased or decreased heart rate

   • Muscle tightness or aches

   • Nausea

   • Queasiness

   • Rigid, tight posture

   • Shakiness

   • Slumped posture

   • Spacey

   • Tearfulness

   • Tight, constricted throat

   • Tingling

   • Weakness

   Notice that the list of bodily sensations above focuses on discomforts and disquieting changes from a normal, relaxed body. When you're feeling positive, happy, or contented, your body's sensations aren't so noticeable. Positive emotions are associated with less easily identified bodily sensations such as rhythmic breathing, relaxed muscles, and an absence of discomfort.

4. **Record your feelings in column two.**

   Try to come up with a feeling word that captures what's going on in your body and mind. Feeling words include

- Angry
- Annoyed
- Anxious
- Apprehensive
- Bitter
- Content
- Dejected
- Despondent
- Distraught
- Embarrassed
- Enthusiastic
- Excited
- Fearful
- Furious
- Gloomy
- Grief
- Guilty
- Happy
- Hopeless
- Insecure
- Irritated
- Joyful
- Miserable
- Morose
- Panicked
- Peaceful
- Rage
- Relaxed
- Remorseful
- Sad
- Upset
- Worried

Notice when you experience uncomfortable bodily sensations, that your feelings are usually negative. It's hard to have a headache, tightness in your chest, and shakiness while feeling peaceful. Tracking the connection between your body and mind can help you become more in touch with your feelings.

5. **In the third column, write down what was happening at the time you first noticed your sensations and feelings.**

   Take time to reflect. Sometimes the event that set everything off is a real happening in your world like noticing how short the day is, getting a traffic ticket, or walking out into bitter cold. Other times, the event is an image or thought that crosses your mind such as thinking about a previous sad holiday experience or missing someone you care about.

Your feelings and bodily sensations don't come out of nowhere. They're triggered by events. Ask yourself what you were doing and what was going on around you when you noticed a difficult feeling. Don't expect yourself to always be able to tie your feelings to a specific event, but usually you can come up with something that set things off. Practice improves your ability to understand where your feelings are coming from.

Seeing a sample of fishing for feelings

Abigail, a college student with SAD, doesn't always know what she's feeling. However, she is able to sense various bodily sensations. Her story illustrates how bodily sensations and feelings can be connected. In Abigail's case, her therapist suggests a way of tying the two together and connecting them to what's happening (events) in her world.

> **Abigail** swears that she'll never take another evening class in winter. She tightens her grip on the wheel as she drives slowly past the metered parking spots. She feels her heart racing. All the spaces close to the lab building are filled. Cars idle, double parked, drivers hoping for the next student to leave. Abigail, already running behind, slides her car into an ice-covered parking lot almost a mile from her first class.

> She pulls her ski cap down low over her head, flips a scarf around her neck, slips on gloves, and heaves her backpack over her shoulder. Getting out of the car, she gasps as the wind takes her breath away. Her nose starts to run but freezes before dripping onto her scarf. "I never get a good parking spot," she complains to herself. "This winter is the worst ever. I'm going to freeze to death before I make it to class. But I'll probably be mugged first by someone in this dark parking lot!"

> It's barely 4:30 p.m., and the sun's already below the horizon. Tears from the cold wind mix with tears of despair as she trudges through dirty mounds of snow. "I can't believe I am stupid enough to think that I can get

my master's degree. I'll never be able to get through the statistics classes. I may as well drop out now."

Abigail began therapy for her depression about two weeks ago. Her therapist diagnosed her with SAD as this is the second winter in a row she has felt this miserable. Her therapist says Abigail has trouble connecting with her feelings and recommends that she fill out a Fishing for Feelings Form. Table 9-1 is what she comes up with.

Table 9-1	Abigail's Fishing for Feelings Form	
Bodily Sensations	*Feelings*	*Events*
Tightness in hands, heart racing	Anxiety and anger	Inability to find a parking spot
Tears	Despair and sadness	An image of failing crossing her mind
Tears	Hopelessness	Walking a mile in the dark and cold

Sifting through Your Thinking

Most people with SAD attribute their misery to the change in seasons. For many, depression arrives in the fall, settles in through the winter, packs up in spring, and leaves in the summer. For them, seasonal shifts appear to cause and cure their depressive symptoms (see Chapter 3 for info on the various causes of SAD).

However, people with SAD also tend to have certain common thoughts about winter, cold, themselves, the world, and the future. In the following sections, you see how SAD thinking can cloud and darken your feelings and moods.

Whining about winter

People who love winter sports generally look forward to snowfall and cold weather. Avid skiers count the days until they're able to hit the slopes. But most people generally prefer warm weather over cold. And for much of the world, the winter not only brings cold temperatures but also shorter days and longer nights. Except for a few night owls out there, most folks prefer longer periods of daylight over darkness.

Bleak thoughts about winter are quite common. And a certain amount of negativity is absolutely normal (we have occasional negative thoughts, too). On the other hand, if you suffer from SAD, your negative thoughts about winter are likely to be more numerous and persistent. That's because depression is a miserable feeling. For SAD sufferers, depression is usually associated with winter. Therefore, not only is winter cold, dark, and dismal, but also it feels even colder, darker, and more dismal when you're depressed.

The relationship between SAD and negative thinking is actually a two-way street. Yes, the more depressed you are, the more your thinking turns negative. And as your thinking becomes more negative, your depression deepens. However, there is good news here. Whichever way the cycle starts, you can improve your moods by changing the way you think.

First, decide what kinds of negative thinking you experience. In the following list, check off which of the following types of negative thoughts concerning winter you've heard rattling around in your brain at one time or another. This quiz about your thoughts about winter helps you start recognizing your negative thoughts. We left room for a few more thoughts at the end of the list if you notice yourself having other dismal thoughts about winter, cold, or dark that aren't on this list.

Here's your checklist:

❑ I can't stand clearing my car's windshield after an ice storm.

❑ I hate sloshing through slush in the winter.

❑ When it's dark outside at 5:00 p.m. or earlier, I feel utterly miserable.

❑ My body can't stand to be cold.

❑ I hate the hassle of heavy coats, boots, and gloves in the winter.

❑ I hate winter so much; I just stay inside.

❑ I can't imagine how anyone could enjoy short days.

❑ There's nothing good about winter.

❑ I never feel rested in the winter.

❑ When I can't go out and enjoy sunshine, I get cabin fever.

❑ I hate socializing in the winter because it's too dark and cold.

❑ I'm terrified of driving in the snow and ice.

❑ _____

❑ _____

❑ _____

Now that you've filled out your quiz (you did fill it out, didn't you?), you may be thinking, what next? The next step is to get a better handle on the other types of negative thoughts that you may have from time to time, especially when you're depressed. That step comes in the next section.

Thinking negatively about yourself

Negative thinking typically accompanies all types of depression. Not only do you have negative thoughts toward winter, darkness, and cold but also thoughts about yourself, too. Therefore, it's important for you to see what negative thoughts about yourself look like.

As with SAD thoughts about winter (preceding section), merely monitoring your thinking sometimes helps those thoughts dissipate (if you want extra help, check out Chapter 10).

Read through the following list of thoughts about yourself. Check off any thoughts that you've experienced, especially during times of low or depressed moods. Go ahead and check an item if it comes close, but doesn't quite capture your actual thoughts because you can also feel free to make a few changes in the words to make them fit your specific ways of thinking. And be sure to add any additional negative thoughts you may have about yourself in the blank lines provided.

Here's the checklist:

❏ I've been eating so much that I feel like a total pig.

❏ I don't care if I have SAD; I'm a lazy slug when I sleep so much.

❏ I don't think I'm as good as other people.

❏ I see myself as inadequate.

❏ I flat out don't like myself.

❏ I regret wasting so much of my life.

❏ I tend to blame myself for almost everything that goes wrong.

❏ I have no self-control at all with candy, carbohydrates, and sweets.

❏ There must be something terribly wrong with me; other people can handle winter.

❏ I'm a terrible person for neglecting my friends.

❏ I am so pathetic when I shut myself up during the dark days.

❏ I am just so ashamed of myself when I can't get moving.

❏ _____

❏ _____

❏ _____

Did any of these thoughts sound familiar? Were you able to come up with additional, negative thoughts that you've noticed in your head? This quiz has no score, and you don't pass or fail. Instead, it's designed to help you see the nature of your negative thoughts about yourself. At the same time, if you checked a lot of these thoughts (more than three or so), it does suggest that consulting a professional may be in order.

Some people actually experience a worsening in their moods when they start tracking their negative thoughts. In essence they experience negative thoughts about the fact that they have negative thoughts in the first place. Please realize that you didn't ask for negative thoughts; they are almost always involved with depression. But if you can't shake a temporary deterioration in your moods, seek professional help. You're likely to still find this book helpful, but a professional consultation is the best idea.

Thinking about the world around you

Every day the news is filled with headlines about wars, starvation, AIDS, crime, torture, corruption, inflation, terrorism, and more. It's no wonder people are depressed. If you pay attention to the misery around you, it may seem reasonable to be sad.

However, people who suffer from SAD often dwell on the negative parts of life instead of seeing at least some of the sunshine. After all, beautiful days, family, kindness, art, caring, and friends all still exist. And hope is still alive. Depressed thinking often involves thinking in terms of all or none. Take Daniel's example:

Daniel, a regional salesman for a software company, is having a tough year. The economy is sluggish, and his regular customers are putting off upgrading their software. As a result, Daniel's sales are down. Plus, he feels constantly tired and is having trouble getting up in the morning. This winter season seems to be stretching out longer than usual, with cold and icy conditions occurring into March.

He goes out with a friend for lunch and finds himself getting more and more agitated as he recounts his woes. "My customers have all stopped buying from me again," he begins. "The stock market hasn't even started to claw its way back. I may lose my house. I've been noticing that the other salespeople in my office are avoiding me."

His buddy is surprised by Daniel's dismal dialogue and attempts to change the subject to something less depressing. He asks Daniel about how his kids are doing. "Well, the school system is horrible. I'm afraid if I leave the kids in public school they'll become juvenile delinquents. But, I can't afford private school because of my terrible sales record," Daniel declares. His friend declines comment and decides to finish his lunch quickly.

Do you tend to make global, all-encompassing statements about the condition of your world? If so, you may be setting yourself up for bad moods. Of course the world isn't all good, but take a look at the following checklist of thoughts about your world as you perceive it:

❑ I don't think there's anyone out there I can trust.

❑ The world is a dangerous place.

❑ People don't like me very much.

❑ People are all out for themselves; it's a dog-eat-dog world.

❑ All politicians are crooks.

❑ There's so much crime out in the world that no one is ever safe.

❑ I can't stand my job.

❑ I hate the hassles of everyday life.

❑ No one can get ahead in today's world.

❑ Life has few pleasures available for me.

❑ I can't count on anyone for help.

❑ I'm overwhelmed by everyday stress in my world.

❑ _____

❑ _____

❑ _____

So, do any of these thoughts describe your outlook on life and the world? Don't be concerned if you have occasional thoughts like these; everyone has them here and there. But if these gloomy perspectives present themselves most of the time, then they contribute to your SAD. Again, like the quiz in the preceding section, there's no pass or fail cutoff point. The purpose of the quiz is to help you understand the types of negative thoughts you tend to have about the world. The blanks are for filling in any specific thoughts you have that weren't covered.

Seeing dark clouds on the horizon

Possibly the most subversive type of negative thinking SAD sufferers can have involves thoughts about the future. People with almost any type of depression look at their future prospects through a pessimistic lens. Rarely do they foresee positive possibilities. Their minds cloud over with thoughts of hopelessness and despair.

Everyone worries about the future. It's normal to have concerns about things like global warming and the future in general. However, if these thoughts dominate your mind, it's hard to get energized to do anything positive. During the winter, people with SAD tend to be pessimistic predictors. They often feel that spring will never arrive, and their world will continue to be dark. Yet, spring will follow winter, the days will be brighter, and you don't have to suffer from SAD year after year.

This problem is big because if you don't see hope for improvement, your motivation is majorly lacking. Fortunately, the very fact that you're reading this book means you likely have at least a smidgeon of hope for a brighter tomorrow.

Here's a checklist to see if you have dismal thoughts about the future:

❑ I can't see anything but a continuing string of depressing winters to come.

❑ I'll never kick this depression.

❑ It's likely that my winter depression will continue through the spring and summer.

❑ There's no hope for peace ever in the world.

❑ I am sure that I won't be able to survive retirement.

❑ Social Security won't exist at all in a few years.

❑ Healthcare will become too expensive for anyone but the very rich.

❑ I anticipate a sad future for myself.

❑ I don't think I'll ever get over my recurring SAD, so why try?

❑ I will probably die sad and alone.

❑ I see myself as hopeless.

❑ _____

❑ _____

❑ _____

This quiz is just like the previous two quizzes. That's right; there's no pass or fail point, and the intent is merely to increase your awareness of the types of negative thoughts you may have about the future.

Tying Together Triggers, Thoughts, and Feelings

Cognitive or thought therapy is an active approach to treating SAD. In order to get better, you need to do a little work. That means filling out exercises and forms as you go along. Don't simply read this book; put it into practice. By the way, no one is going to check up on you for spelling and grammar. And we tried to make the work interesting.

Discovering the SAD Thought Tracker

Begin tracking your feelings (and associated bodily sensations), thoughts, and events that started your negative thoughts. You can do this on a SAD Thought Tracker.

Here's how a SAD Thought Tracker works:

1. **Pull out a notebook (or copy the form in Appendix A) and draw three columns with headings:** *Feelings and Sensations, Events,* **and** *Thoughts or Interpretations.*

2. **In the first column,** *Feelings and Sensations,* **write down both your body's sensations and a feeling word that describes those sensations.**

   Look back at the section "Fishing for Feelings" earlier in this chapter for guidance. Also rate the feeling words for intensity from 1 (very mild) to 100 (extremely intense or severe). You may have more than one feeling and/or sensations. Write them all here and rate the feeling.

3. **In the second column,** *Events,* **write down what you think may have triggered the feelings and sensations from Step 2.**

   Ask yourself what was going on. Usually events involve something that happens to you. But sometimes, what gets everything rolling is a day-dream or an image that floats into your mind.

4. **In the last column,** *Thoughts or Interpretations,* **record your thoughts about the event from Step 3.**

   Thoughts reflect the meaning or interpretation you have about what happened. It's common to have difficulty in figuring out what your thoughts are about events that happen. The following questions may help you figure out what you think about what has occurred:

- What just passed through my mind when the event happened?

- What does this happening say about me as a person?

- How will this event affect my future?

- What's the worst thing about this event?

- How will this event affect my life today?

- How am I interpreting or what meaning am I making out of this event?

Seeing a SAD Thought Tracker in action

SAD can creep up unexpectedly. Sometimes your life can seem like it just starts spiraling out of control and you have no good idea as to what's going on. Thought trackers can help you get a handle on the issues.

The family in the following story illustrates how thought trackers can help clarify the relationship between everyone's feelings, events, and thoughts or interpretations. Gathering that information can lead to productive actions.

Ted, his wife **Kathleen,** and teenage daughter **Lisa,** relocate from Phoenix, Arizona, to Portland, Oregon. Ted works for a computer chip manufacturer and is transferred. Kathleen has no trouble getting a job as a special education teacher, and Lisa transfers into the sophomore class at the local high school. The family misses the sunny Arizona days, but the move is very good financially. The family enjoys cycling in the mild Portland summer. But trouble is brewing.

As the school year begins, Lisa seems to be unhappy and unenthusiastic. Kathleen and Ted think that it's likely the adjustment to the new school. They agree to give it some more time. Ted and Lisa start arguing all the time. Ted is constantly nagging Lisa to do her homework and get off the phone. Kathleen tries to intervene but isn't able to help. Life just doesn't seem as good as it used to be.

Kathleen is stunned when she opens Lisa's report card for the fall semester. Lisa was always a good student, and the failing grades are totally unexpected. When confronted, Lisa becomes uncharacteristically angry. Ted arrives home and hears about the grades — he explodes, and the family erupts. Doors slam, and Ted launches into a tirade. Kathleen wonders what is happening to their previously peaceful family.

Fortunately, Ted, Kathleen, and Lisa all agree to start family counseling. Their psychologist determines that they're all depressed and may be suffering from SAD although further depression in coming years would be needed for the diagnosis to be definitive (see Chapter 2). The therapist brings up the stress of the recent move and suggests that each member of the family complete a few SAD Thought Trackers. They can use this information to compare how they're all thinking and perhaps come up with some solutions. Their thoughts are in Tables 9-2, 9-3, and 9-4.

Table 9-2	Ted's SAD Thought Tracker	
Feelings and Sensations	*Events*	*Thoughts or Interpretations*
Overwhelming sadness, I feel very tired (95). I feel really sad and lethargic.	Moving to Portland	This mistake was horrible. I never should've moved; I've hurt my family. The weather is utterly awful.
Anger and irritation (75). I feel jittery and helpless.	Fighting with my daughter Lisa	She's spoiled. She has everything she wants. All I ask for is decent grades.
Anger and disappointment (80). I don't know what to do, and that bothers me.	Lisa's bad grades	I work so hard. How can Lisa do this to me? I must be a terrible father.

Table 9-3	Kathleen's SAD Thought Tracker	
Feelings and Sensations	*Events*	*Thoughts or Interpretations*
Excited and happy (80)	Moving to Portland	This move is a great career move for me. I'll finally be able to start my graduate degree.
Depressed (90). I just start crying every time they fight.	Ted and Lisa fighting	My husband and daughter must hate each other. I feel stuck in the middle.
Anger and disappointment (75). Tense, shallow breathing	Lisa's bad grades	Lisa isn't happy. This situation is my fault. I was too concerned about my own career. I'm not a good mother.

Table 9-4	Lisa's SAD Thought Tracker	
Feelings and Sensations	*Events*	*Thoughts or Interpretations*
Grief and loss (100). Overwhelming fatigue	Moving to Portland	I'll never get over leaving all my friends. I can't stand Portland; it rains all the time.
Anger (90). Racing heart beat and tightness in my chest	Arguing with my dad	He doesn't understand. All he cares about is his stupid job.
Hopeless (85). Constantly tired	My bad grades	It's not that I can't do the work; I just want to spend the day in bed. I feel so stupid. I just want to drop out of school.

Ted, Kathleen, and Lisa look over each other's SAD Thought Trackers. They are rather surprised to see that they're all feeling miserable and having dark, bleak thoughts. For the first time in months, the family gathers and comforts each other. They vow to get the help they need and spend more positive family time together.

Detecting Distortions in SAD Thinking

A basic premise of thought therapy is the idea that the way you think about or interpret events, greatly influences how you feel. The section "Tying Together Triggers, Thoughts, and Feelings" shows you those connections. The examples showed that the characters uniformly expressed thoughts that were negative and dismal.

In this section, we show you specific ways in which most negative thoughts in response to happenings are distorted. Distorted thoughts contain inaccuracies, misinterpretations, and flawed descriptions of events. These inaccuracies cause you to feel worse than you need to.

When you first jot your thoughts or interpretations of events down on paper, you probably won't instantly notice these inaccuracies. In fact, you're more likely to believe that your thoughts pretty much reflect the way things are. But as you examine the various ways in which thoughts can be distorted, you're likely to start seeing what we're talking about. Figuring out how to detect thought distortions actually can be a little fun and certainly can put you on a path toward recovery.

We've searched high and low and never run into a single person who doesn't occasionally have distorted thoughts. Everyone from time to time sees things as worse, more awful, or more dire than they really are. This situation happens more frequently when people are tired, hungry, irritable, sad, anxious, or in some other negative state of mind. Depressed folks just happen to engage in distorted thinking with increased frequency and intensity. However, even if you've never been depressed, understanding how to capture your distorted thoughts and remolding them to more accurately reflect what's going on can improve your outlook and state of mind.

We call distortions in thinking *reality scramblers*. In our work with SAD patients, we see two major types of reality scramblers: The information reality scramblers and the judging reality scramblers.

The information reality scramblers

The information reality scramblers describe the various ways the mind has of twisting your interpretations of information that comes to you. These scramblers can make events seem downright awful. Thus your mood is likely to feel pretty low as well.

For example, if the weather turns cold, someone with SAD is likely to think, "I can't stand terrible weather. The hassles with the car are just unbelievable — scraping the windshield, driving in the snow, waiting forever for the engine to warm up. I just hate winter!" These thoughts contain a number of information reality scramblers covered in the following sections.

If a person didn't use reality scramblers, the thoughts may sound more like, "I really don't like bad weather; it's kind of a hassle messing with scraping the windshield and waiting for the car to warm up. This isn't my favorite time of year." Can you see how this kind of thinking is likely to lead to less severe emotional reactions to the weather?

Please be aware that the various information reality scramblers in the next sections can overlap with each other. That's okay. We list them all separately because it helps people to know the various forms that these scramblers come in. Don't worry about memorizing the list or always knowing exactly which one applies to your thoughts. Sometimes a given thought will involve more than one information reality scrambler.

Awfulizing

This scrambler is pretty easy to detect. Generally speaking, when you think of something as downright *awful,* you're probably interpreting things as worse than they really are. For example, some people with SAD think that snow storms are truly "awful." Many events in life are truly unpleasant, disagreeable, or a little distressing. However, most of the time when you declare them as awful, your mind is tricking you into a significant distortion of the reality.

Exaggeration

Depressed minds have a tendency to exaggerate or enlarge the importance of unpleasant or bad events. For example, someone with SAD may have the thought that a small mistake leads to the loss of her job. The next time you're upset by something, try asking yourself how important the event will be in a week or a month. If it seems it will be much less important, you were probably exaggerating that event in your mind.

Personalizing

This reality scrambler transforms events or circumstances that aren't really about you into something that's about you. For example, someone cuts you off in traffic, and you interpret the maneuver as an aggressive act aimed at you personally. Or, your spouse comes home upset about being overworked, and you assume that she's mad at you.

All-or-none thinking

Few things in life are completely good or totally bad; most events have many shades of gray. However, this information reality scrambler applies an all-or-none, black-and-white set of standards. Thus any instance of a less-than-stellar performance or outcome is viewed as a complete and total failure. People who use this scrambler often think that if they aren't perfect in every way, then they're totally worthless. This case is never true of anyone!

Negative predicting

This reality scrambler looks at the future and predicts disaster, gloom, and doom. Facts aren't relevant. Usually, there's no reason for anticipating bad outcomes. For example, you hear the weather forecast for the week, which says it will be sunny, but you're certain it will rain every day.

Dismissing evidence

Sometimes evidence comes your way that may be able to tell you that all is actually well in your world, at least for the moment. However, you dismiss the evidence and toss the information aside. For example, imagine that you're a new struggling artist who just received a great review in a national newspaper for your work. Instead of thinking how this can help your career, you choose to believe that reviews mean nothing in the art world and that your work will never really sell.

Can't stand its

People say "I can't stand it" so often that it can begin to sound like a song you can't get out of your mind like "It's a Small World After All . . ." (sorry if that got you going). This information scrambler makes you think that something is so horrible that you may actually die or go nuts. For example, you may think that you can't stand winter and cold weather, but odds are you won't die. In our experience, there are loads of things people *don't like,* but very few that they actually *can't stand.*

Filtering

SAD minds quite often seek out negative information while completely screening out the positive. When you apply that filter to yourself and the world, everything looks quite bleak indeed. For example, someone with SAD may receive a job evaluation containing 15 positive statements and two small, negative items. The conclusion? "I'm a complete failure."

Mind reading

This information reality scrambler causes you to make assumptions about other people's thoughts and reactions. In other words, you just *know* what people think about you. Like all the scramblers, the assumptions are negative and gloomy. So, you think, "I won't ask for a raise because I know my boss doesn't like me."

Minimizing

This method of distorting reality takes a look at positive outcomes and minimizes them, thereby robbing you of a chance to feel good about something for a change. For example, if you see 14 copies of the various *For Dummies* books you wrote in the bookstore, you may compare your shelf-space to a former President or famous TV psychologist who has far more copies of his books on display.

Overgeneralizing

This reality scrambler involves noticing one instance of a poor or negative outcome and making the assumption that the event actually represents an unending string of future disasters to come. Thus, if you make one bad decision on a stock purchase, you may begin thinking, "I'm an idiot who always makes poor choices. I never think things through well enough."

Be on the lookout for the words *always* and *never* in your thoughts. They can tip you off that you may be *overgeneralizing.*

Here come the judging reality scramblers

People with SAD carry a harsh critic around on their shoulders. This judge makes swift, cruel decisions without careful consideration of the facts. The gavel slams down along with declarations such as, "You're guilty," "You should have known better," or "You're a despicable human being!" Does any of this sound familiar? The judging reality scramblers come in four major forms. Although each scrambler has a fairly clear definition, they actually overlap quite a bit. Most thoughts generally contain more than one scrambler at a time. In fact, some SAD thoughts contain quite a few! Each scrambler is covered in the following sections.

Self-blame

This judging reality scrambler finds ways of blaming you for all that goes wrong. This scrambler isn't about failing to take a reasonable degree of responsibility for bad happenings; rather, self-blame is about accusing yourself of heinous intentions and criminal negligence when bad things occur. For example, one of your stock purchases tumbles by 50 percent overnight after a bad news report. Although the report could not have been anticipated, you conclude that you were an idiot for having made the purchase.

Shoulding

Who doesn't say, "I should have . . . ?" Everyone does. But when *should* litters your thoughts like trash along the side of a neglected highway, you're probably under the influence of a reality scrambler. Shoulding isn't the same as assessing an action to understand how to do something better the next time; it's about trashing all you've done as never being good enough.

Critical comparisons

It's so easy to pummel yourself with this scrambler. No human is ever the most perfectly attractive, talented, intelligent, kind, or successful person in the world. Even the most beautiful or handsome movie stars aren't perfectly beautiful or handsome 24 hours a day, 7 days a week. When you engage in critical comparisons, you put yourself down by finding examples of others who you believe are better than you.

Self-tagging

Most of us don't go around calling other people stupid, clumsy, crazy, or pathetic. It isn't polite. Calling names is just not nice. But when people are depressed, they all too frequently tag themselves with such labels. A SAD sufferer may think such things as, "I'm a fat pig for eating so much;" "I'm lazy when I sleep so late;" or "I must be stupid when I can't concentrate." Someone without SAD would typically think, "I ate a little too much," "Looks like I overslept!" or "I feel a little distracted today."

Recording reality scramblers on SAD Thought Trackers

Distorted thinking is a habit. And habits are hard to break. Giving up scrambled thinking is a little like quitting smoking. You may find it easy to quit . . .

again and again and again. So, be patient and practice. But keep in mind that practice doesn't make perfect; practice just makes it better. The goal is progress, not perfection, so take it one day at a time.

Record your reality scrambler as follows:

1. **In a notebook, divide a page into four columns (or copy the SAD Thought Tracker pages in Appendix A).**

2. **In the first column, write down your feelings and sensations.**

3. **In column 2, jot down a description of what happened or what went through your mind.**

4. **In the third column, briefly describe your thoughts.**

5. **Read through the list of reality scramblers in the two sections above and see whether any of them fit your situations.**

   Think about how the scrambler may have disturbed you or increased your depression and write the scramblers in the fourth column. In Chapter 10, you see how to scrape away scramblers and clean up your thinking.

In the section "Tying Together Triggers, Thoughts, and Feelings," you met Ted, Kathleen, and Lisa, a family that moved from Phoenix to Portland and began to have problems with SAD. Tracking their thoughts helped them understand and deal with what was happening. Tables 9-5 through 9-7 give you some examples of their completed SAD Thought Trackers with the reality scramblers added.

Table 9-5	Ted's SAD Thought Tracker and Reality Scramblers		
Feelings	*Events*	*Thoughts*	*Reality Scramblers*
Overwhelming sadness. I feel very tired (95). I feel really sad and lethargic.	Moving to Portland	This mistake was horrible. I should've never moved. I've hurt my family. The weather is utterly awful.	Exaggeration, shoulding, self-blame, awfulizing
Anger and irritation (75). I feel jittery and helpless.	Fighting with my daughter Lisa	She's spoiled. She has everything she wants. All I ask for is decent grades.	Exaggeration, overgeneralizing, filtering
Anger and disappointment (80). I don't know what to do, and that bothers me.	Lisa's bad grades	I work so hard. How can Lisa do this to me? I must be a terrible father.	Personalizing, self-tagging

Table 9-6   Kathleen's SAD Thought Tracker and Reality Scramblers

Feelings	Events	Thoughts	Reality Scramblers
Excited and happy (80).	Moving to Portland	This move is a great career move for me. I'll finally be able to start my graduate degree.	None
Depressed (90). I just start crying every time they fight.	Ted and Lisa fighting	My husband and daughter must hate each other. I feel stuck in the middle.	Mind reading, exaggeration
Anger and disappointment (75). Tense, shallow breathing	Lisa's bad grades	Lisa isn't happy. This situation is my fault. I was too concerned about my own career. I'm not a good mother.	Self-tagging, self-blame

Table 9-7   Lisa's SAD Thought Tracker and Reality Scramblers

Feelings	Events	Thoughts	Reality Scramblers
Grief and loss (100). Overwhelming fatigue	Moving to Portland	I'll never get over leaving all my friends. I can't stand Portland; it rains all of the time.	Negative predicting, overgeneralizing, all-or-none thinking, can't stand its
Anger (90). Racing heart beat and tightness in my chest	Arguing with my dad	He doesn't understand. All he cares about is his stupid job.	Mind reading, filtering
Hopeless (85). Constantly tired	My bad grades	It's not that I can't do the work; I just want to spend the day in bed. I feel so stupid. I just want to drop out of school.	Self-tagging, exaggerating

Quizzing Your SAD Reality Scramblers

SAD is a type of depression. Everyone who's depressed scrambles reality in similar, depressing ways. Things seem worse than they are, problems appear insurmountable, and the future looks grim. However, people with SAD also tend to use scramblers in how they view winter, cold, and dark.

See Table 9-8 for examples of depressive thinking related to SAD. See if you can figure out which reality scramblers are at work. Don't stress out over this exercise! The answers come after the table.

Table 9-8	SAD Thought Tracker and Reality Scramblers		
Feelings	*Events*	*Thoughts*	*Reality Scramblers*
Miserable (80) anxiety and tension	Turning the clocks back in the fall	I can't stand it when it's dark at 4:30 p.m.	
Tension, tightness in chest. Anxiety (90)	A cold snap hits.	There's nothing worse than winter. My car probably won't start, and I'll be late to work tomorrow.	
Stomach in knots, spacey, disoriented. Hopeless (80)	An ice storm cuts off electricity.	I bet I lost everything on my computer. I'm probably going to freeze all night. This winter will never end — it's awful.	
Hunger pangs, constricted muscles, shivering. Stressed and unhappy (70)	Walking from the parking garage to the mall in the bitter cold.	I shouldn't have come to the mall tonight. I'm so stupid. I have to find something to eat; I'm starving.	

Here are Table 9-8's results:

- ✔ In the first event (turning back the clocks), the thoughts showed evidence of the *can't stand its* reality scrambler.

- ✔ The second event (cold weather), induced thoughts that were scrambled by *all-or-none thinking* and *negative predicting*.

- ✔ The third example (ice storm) created thoughts with *exaggeration, negative predicting,* and *awfulizing*.

- ✔ The final event (walking from the parking garage to the mall) demonstrated thoughts that were riddled by *shoulding, self-tagging,* and *exaggerating*.

Chapter 10

Brightening Up SAD Thinking

*R*ight now, our dog Murphy is leaping, barking, and jumping at our back-yard window. Thinking she's protecting us, she growls at a couple of guys who've spent the last eight days working on a project that we think should've taken about six hours. Each hour they stay costs us more money. Every once in a while, one of them wants to come in and use the bathroom. When they do, Murphy runs around in circles, and our other dog, Joey, normally quiet, joins in the fracas.

We work at home. It has been a bad writing day. We're starting to feel anxious, stressed, and down. We're having thoughts like, "We'll never finish this book;" "The dogs are driving us insane;" "We should have checked out these workers more carefully;" "We're so stupid to have to pay so much for this project;" "Why did we ever take on another book project?"

But you know what? We're cognitive therapists. We've educated ourselves on how to catch such thinking and turn it around.

There are two major categories of thought change strategies:

> ✔ The first category involves using *logic* and *gathering evidence* to change the way you look at things.

> ✔ The second category is called *emotional distancing*. After you've stepped back, it's easier to change your viewpoint and find better ways of thinking about events.

In this chapter, we show you how to change your thinking. You discover how to take your thoughts, track them carefully, and revise them in ways that make you feel better.

Listening to Logic and Evidence

When you feel sad, hopeless, and depressed, you may not want to hear the message — get logical. The feeling of depression can be so intense and so painful, that looking for evidence as a way to feel better seems sort of silly and almost meaningless. And you probably believe that your thoughts are absolutely true and accurately reflect the depressing state of affairs you find yourself in.

But guess what? Numerous studies show that looking at evidence and logic to straighten out thinking can reduce the effects of seasonal affective disorder (SAD). It works. To make this approach more appealing, think in terms of the popular CSI (crime scene investigators) shows on TV. In the TV programs, the investigators are presented with a crime scene, or the end result or a series of circumstances. Often, what seems obvious as the cause behind the end result isn't the case at all. It is only through applying logic and reason to the evidence that the truth emerges.

In the following sections, you discover techniques that use logic, reasoning, and evidence to change depressive, distorted, or scrambled thoughts. Try them out yourself to see how these strategies can loosen up your thinking and improve your mood. You can be a little skeptical at first, but do open up your mind to the possibility that this approach helps. So, put on your detective hat and take a closer look.

Unscrambling reality scramblers

If you read Chapter 9, you uncovered the various ways that thoughts can be scrambled or distorted. In that chapter, you figure out ways for detecting whether your thoughts have any of these reality scramblers. But *this* chapter is about discovering how to *change* your thinking. For the sake of convenience, so you don't have to flip back and forth to Chapter 9, the major types of reality scramblers are listed in Table 10-1. Be sure to look at Chapter 9 if you want more info and complete definitions of reality scramblers.

Table 10-1	Types of Reality Scramblers
Distortion	*Definition*
All-or-none thinking	The world is full of grays, but this distortion makes you think in black and white terms. Thus, you may conclude that a single imperfection means you're nothing at all.
Awfulizing	When you think about something as truly awful, you're probably using this distortion because few things are truly awful and horrible.

Distortion	*Definition*
Can't stand its	Many unpleasant events in life occur but very few that you truly "can't stand." When you say you can't stand something, you probably make yourself more miserable than you need to.
Critical comparisons	This distortion occurs when you frequently compare yourself, your work, your accomplishments, and so on to others who may be somewhat better at one thing or another.
Dismissing evidence	Sometimes good things happen even to people who are depressed! But this distortion makes you think that evidence about positive possibilities actually means nothing.
Exaggeration	This reality scrambler applies to all the ways your mind exaggerates the importance and unpleasantness of events.
Filtering	Whenever you ignore the good events and focus on negative, you use the filtering scrambler.
Mind reading	If you discover yourself making gloomy conclusions about other people's opinions, thoughts, or reactions, you're mind reading if there's no strong evidence to support your automatic negative assumption.
Minimizing	This scrambler looks at positive information or feedback and minimizes it.
Negative predicting	If you're a diehard pessimist who always expects the worst, you probably use this reality scrambler.
Overgeneralizing	This scrambler involves looking at one bad occurrence and concluding that it simply foretells a series of similar events.
Personalizing	This scrambler occurs when your mind concludes that an event was aimed at you even though the evidence fails to support that conclusion.
Self-blame	When things go wrong, it's actually healthy to accept a reasonable degree of responsibility. However, self-blame assigns *all* blame to yourself, giving rise to feelings of worthlessness.
Self-tagging	This scrambler searches for disgusting labels to put on yourself. Calling yourself lazy, stupid, or fat doesn't help matters.
Shoulding	This scrambler works when you scold yourself by saying you "should" have done things differently or "should" have known better.

A reality scrambler is similar to someone using a ruse at a crime scene to misdirect the investigation. Your job, should you accept the assignment, is to collect and sort through the evidence to uncover what's really going on. The good news is that, unlike on the CSI shows where the crime is solved but the victim doesn't leave the morgue, unscrambling thought scramblers can breathe new light and life into your attitude and outlook.

Examples provide a great way to acquire a new skill. So, take a look at how Ethan collected evidence and applied logic to unscramble his thought scramblers:

> **Ethan,** a 30-something electrical engineer living in Chicago, breaks up with his girlfriend of five years. The breakup is difficult for Ethan, but he's also a little relieved. She was quite irritable and difficult to please, but Ethan stayed with her in part out of habit. He's eager to find another relationship because he enjoys having a steady companion.
>
> A few months go by, and Ethan is becoming anxious. It seems like all the nicer women around him are taken. He's not sure how to meet anyone and is afraid of online dating services. He becomes pessimistic about his situation.
>
> A cold Chicago winter blows into town. The sky is steel gray, and darkness closes in early. Ethan finds himself eating more and going out less. He realizes that his work suffers. He lacks enthusiasm and ambition. Many people have symptoms of SAD in Chicago during the winter. Ethan picks up a copy of *Seasonal Affective Disorder For Dummies* and completes the SAD Thought Tracker and Reality Unscrambler Exercise in Table 10-2. See Chapter 9 for more examples of SAD Thought Trackers.

Table 10-2	Ethan's SAD Thought Tracker and Reality Unscrambler Exercise	
Feelings and Sensations	*Events*	*Thoughts or Interpretations*
Sullen and despondent (88), tense muscles	Not having a date for the company holiday party.	I'll never find anyone.
Hopeless (75), no energy	Went to a lunch event for singles and didn't connect with anyone.	I'm a total loser. I can tell immediately that none of the women like me.
Shivering, discomfort, and anxiety (80)	Walking home from the subway.	I can't stand weather like this. And when the sun goes down so early, it's downright awful.

Initial Thoughts	Reality Scramblers	Unscrambled Thoughts
I'll never find anyone.	Negative predicting, overgeneralizing	I didn't find anyone at this party, but that doesn't mean anything about the future.
I'm a total loser. I can tell immediately that none of the women like me.	Self-tagging, overgeneralizing, mind reading	Calling myself a loser just makes me feel bad and doesn't help. I really don't know how the women feel about me. I think I may be giving out negative vibes.
I can't stand weather like this. And when the sun goes down so early, it's downright awful.	Awfulizing, can't stand its, exaggeration	Winter weather in Chicago does sort of stink, but I can stand it. I don't like it when it gets dark early, but it isn't horrible or awful. I really need to remember to wear gloves and maybe get some better lighting for my apartment. I can do something about these things.

Rating the results:

After looking at the Unscrambled Thoughts section, I do feel a little better. My sullenness and despondence has gone down to about a 65; I don't feel so hopeless now; it's down to about 25. And anxiety about the weather is about a 40; I guess I really can stand it. I can see where this exercise actually helped a little. I'm feeling more optimistic. I think I'll keep doing this for a while.

So Ethan figured out that his negative thoughts usually contained significant distortions in the form of various reality scramblers. By seeing those scramblers in action, he was able to rethink things in a more logical, reasonable manner. His feelings improved as a result.

Feel fee to make copies of the SAD Thought Tracker and Reality Unscrambler Form in Appendix A to help you unscramble your thinking. Here are the directions for filling out your own SAD Thought Tracker and Reality Unscrambler Form (refer to Table 10-2 for help):

1. **In the first column, *Feelings and Sensations*, write down both your body's sensations and a feeling word that describes those sensations.**

   Also rate the feeling words for intensity from 1 (very mild) to 100 (extremely intense or severe). Thus, 25 represents a noticeable, but fairly mild level; 50 indicates significant intensity, but not overwhelming, 75 suggests that the feeling is pretty intense, and 100 would be overwhelming.

2. **In the second column, *Events,* write down what you think may have triggered the feelings and sensations, and ask yourself what was going on.**

3. **In the last column, *Thoughts,* record your thoughts about the event.**

   Thoughts reflect the meaning or interpretation you have about what happened.

4. **Briefly rewrite your initial thoughts from the SAD Thought Tracker in the column labeled *Initial Thoughts.***

5. **Refer to the Reality Scrambler list in Table 10-1 and jot down any reality scramblers under *Reality Scramblers* that you believe may be contained within your thoughts.**

6. **Write down thoughts that express a more realistic, less scrambled perspective on your initial thoughts in the column labeled *Unscrambled Thoughts.***

7. **Finally, rate your results.**

   In other words, take another look at your feelings and indicate whether they've changed. Express what you feel you got out of the exercise. See Table 10-2 for a finalized example.

The change strategies in this chapter usually take some practice — typically it helps to continue doing them for a number of weeks. And don't think that your first shot at them will make everything better. Sometimes you will struggle with these exercises. Working with a mental health professional can provide an important boost and additional support. After you thoroughly study and practice these strategies, they become part of your new way of thinking.

Positively true

A common misunderstanding about cognitive therapy is the belief that its goal is to persuade you to think positively all the time. And if you actually thought that was the goal of this approach, it would be reasonable for you to balk at trying this therapy out. You might say, "I don't want to be delusional! I want to see things as they are."

We agree completely. Cognitive therapists want you to know how to view yourself, the world, the future, and the seasons in realistic, objective terms. We want you to see things pretty much as they are. We don't believe in sugar coating and trying to see the world through rose-colored glasses. That's because sometimes bad and sad events do happen, and it's important to acknowledge them and take appropriate actions for dealing with misfortune when it does occur. For example, in many places it really gets bitter cold in the winter, and darkness arrives earlier than most people like. But there are useful things you can do about these conditions.

Collecting evidence about thoughts

In the beginning of this chapter, we were griping about our dogs, the slow pace of the work in our backyard, and all the interruptions. When we write books, we generally run a pretty tight schedule. So, unexpected interruptions can really put us behind. Then the other day we had tickets to return to New Mexico, and it snowed several inches, which gridlocked the Albuquerque airport and stranded us for hours and hours in the Las Vegas, Nevada, airport.

It's hard to write a book in any airport, but in Vegas it's impossible with the blaring announcements, greetings, general chaos, and the clinging, buzzing, and obnoxious noises of hundreds of slot machines. After attempting to rebook our flight, find our luggage, book a hotel, and wait for a shuttle — we were exhausted. That night at dinner we had the following conversation:

> **Chuck:** This situation is so frustrating. We stood around looking for our luggage for more than two hours! A few inches of snow and the whole state shuts down? I hate winter.
>
> **Laura:** I can't believe we wasted an entire day at this airport. It's driving me crazy. And when we get home we have to drive on slippery highways with New Mexico drivers. Ugh.
>
> **Chuck:** And do you realize how far behind we are on this book? We'll never catch up.
>
> **Laura:** I can't believe that we agreed to this again.
>
> **Chuck:** All we do is work.
>
> **Laura:** Maybe we can skip Christmas dinner and just write.
>
> **Chuck:** That's a great idea. I'm glad we already turned down that party on New Years.
>
> **Laura:** We'll never catch up.
>
> **Chuck:** Hmm, our thinking is turning pretty nasty isn't it?
>
> **Laura:** Yep. Maybe it's time for a dose of our own medicine. Let's *Check the Evidence.*
>
> **Chuck:** I hate it when you're right . . .

Even trained professionals can allow circumstances to cloud and confuse their thinking! So we jotted down how we were feeling, the events connected to those feelings, and the thoughts the feelings and events generated (see Table 10-3). That was our evidence. Next, we applied logic, using these five questions:

✔ Can we think of experiences from our pasts that would contradict these thoughts?

✔ Have we had thoughts like this in the past that didn't prove to be true?

✔ Would we see this issue differently if we were in better moods or if it were summer?

✔ Are there other explanations we haven't considered?

✔ Are we overlooking evidence that would refute our thoughts?

After answering these five questions, we reinterpreted our thoughts based on the evidence, then rated the results of our assessments, and felt much better. Table 10-3 illustrates our process.

Table 10-3	Chuck and Laura's SAD Thought Tracker and Collecting the Evidence Form	
Feelings and Sensations	**Events**	**Thoughts or Interpretations**
Frustrated (80), tense, achy, and tired	Air flight was cancelled; our luggage was lost	This situation is horrible. The whole day was wasted.
Panicky (90), anxious (70), stomach in knots	Realizing that another writing day went down the tubes.	We'll never finish this book! It'll be impossible to meet our deadlines.
Sad (65), hopeless (40), tired	Working too much and deadlines looming.	All we ever do is work. We don't spend enough time with our families.
Initial Thoughts	**Evidence-Based Thoughts (After Asking 5 Questions)**	
This situation is horrible. The whole day was wasted.	Okay, maybe the day was unpleasant. Very unpleasant. But it wasn't "horrible." And we did get a few things accomplished. Chuck got a lot of e-mail caught up, and Laura finished reading a few articles.	
We'll never finish this book! It'll be impossible to meet our deadlines.	We've fallen behind before and we always catch up. Always. (So stop worrying, editor!)	
All we ever do is work. We don't spend enough time with our families.	While we do work a lot, we do enjoy it. We've been spending more time with our families lately in spite of this book. And we can make this whole episode a little more fun by writing about it.	

Rating the Results:

After looking at our evidence-based thoughts, we can see we were getting into a negative spiral of thinking. Our frustration decreased to about 30, we no longer feel panicked, and we're a little sad about missing out on a writing day, but we know we can make it up soon.

You may be thinking, "How can I ever get my thoughts undistorted when a couple of psychologists still think so negatively?" Well, *all* people have negative thoughts, but people who suffer with SAD take their negative thoughts more seriously, have more trouble letting go of them, and often resist changing them. We showed you an example of our negative thinking so you can see that some negative thinking is normal.

Carry around a 3-x-5-inch card with the five evidence-gathering questions on it. That way, it's easy to pull out and review. Work on the collecting the evidence exercise for 10 or 15 minutes on days that you're depressed (and for some weeks after you're no longer depressed). The exercise works much better when you write your thoughts down — don't try to do it in your head. After many practices it becomes the way you think most of the time.

Calculating a cost/benefit analysis

Sometimes people resist letting go of their distorted negative thinking because they believe that their thoughts are beneficial. For example, a committed pessimist may feel that her predictions of gloom and doom prevent her from being disappointed when bad things happen. Or a perfectionist who feels horrible about every single mistake believes he benefits from his perfectionist thoughts because they push him to do his utter best all the time.

In fact, negative thoughts *do* sometimes bestow a few advantages for you! For example, if your blood pressure has been up recently, it is reasonable to have a negative thought in the form of worry about your health. And if that worry causes you to go to the doctor to check it out, then your thought is playing a positive function for you. But typically, with negative thoughts, the disadvantages far outweigh the advantages. So conduct a careful cost/benefit analysis of your negative thinking to assess the pros and cons of each thought.

Here's an example of how to do a cost/benefit analysis with your thoughts:

> **Diana,** lives in a small condo outside of New York City. Her commute is about three hours. On a good day. When it snows, the journey stretches to four or five hours. Today, the train crawls. The car is uncomfortable. People are wet from melting snow, tired from the long day, and crabby. Diana wonders why she ever bought that condo so far away from the city. She thinks, "I am really stupid about money. I always make terrible decisions."

She first uses the SAD Thought Tracker (see Chapter 9 and the section in this chapter on Unscrambling Reality Scramblers for more examples of SAD Thought Trackers) and takes her thoughts from that form to put on her cost/benefit analysis. When she turns to her cost/benefit analysis, at first she thinks, "This is hard. How could those thoughts possibly help me?" But after a little more thought, she comes up with the information in Table 10-4:

Table 10-4	Diana's Cost/Benefit Analysis
Thought: I am really stupid about money. I always make terrible decisions.	
Benefits	**Costs**
When I think this way, I don't disappoint myself. I just accept the status quo. It's easier to complain about something than to do something about it.	This kind of thinking doesn't lead to solving my problems. If I think differently, then maybe I could be proactive and talk to my boss about changing my schedule. Someone else in my office works four ten-hour days.
If I think I'm stupid, then I don't have to take responsibility for my mistakes.	Again, I don't take responsibility for fixing something that isn't working out. If I always make stupid mistakes and terrible decisions, then I'll just be passive and let other people make my decisions. That won't get me where I want to be.
	Thinking this way ends up just making me feel worse in the long run. And doing something about my problems and mistakes isn't all that hard to do.
Rating the results:	
After looking at my cost/benefit analysis I can see that my negative thinking keeps me from solving my problems. I just complain and feel like a victim. I don't have to do that anymore. My feelings of despair now have gone from around 85 to 35. I feel much better.	

As you can see, while Diana's negative thinking yielded a couple of benefits, the costs they were extracting were higher. Although her thinking allowed her to complain without doing any work, she realized that taking responsibility for figuring out solutions would get her where she wants to go more effectively.

Here's how to make your own cost/benefits analysis:

1. **Jot down your initial thought from your SAD Thought Tracker in your notebook.**

2. **In column one, under *Benefits,* start by writing down every conceivable advantage that your negative thought may have for you in the left-hand column.**

   Some people find this part pretty easy; for others, it takes a little thought. If you're in the latter group, you may think at first that your thoughts couldn't possibly help you. But ponder how they can protect you from disappointment, hurt, failure, and so on. Or ask yourself how they might motivate you or help you get what you want.

3. **In the right-hand column, *Costs,* jot down every way that your thought also costs you something, causes you harm, or prevents you from getting what you want.**

   In this column, you can also include reasons why items in the benefit column may not hold water.

4. **Finally rate your results.**

   Jot down how your feelings may have changed. Have your emotions quelled a little and did you benefit from the exercise?

This simple technique clarifies thinking and illuminates unhelpful, negative thoughts. We also like to use the cost/benefit analysis with our clients to help them make decisions about all sorts of issues. See Appendix A for a copy of the Cost/Benefit Analysis Form that you can use. It's also a great strategy to use when you feel conflicted about an important decision such as accepting a job offer, breaking up a relationship, or whether to move.

Putting on a lab coat

Another technique using evidence and logic is called *Checking Thoughts Out.* In effect, this strategy shows you how to go out and collect new evidence as you test your thoughts out in the real world. This technique involves collecting data to verify or refute your negative thinking and requires you to actively solicit information from others.

Some people find that this exercise causes intense anxiety. If that's the case with you, don't do it right now! Instead, consider enlisting the support of a therapist. You might also find it useful to read and work through one of our other books: *Overcoming Anxiety For Dummies* and/or *Anxiety and Depression Workbook For Dummies* (Wiley).

Read the example below to see how checking thoughts out can clear up muddied thinking:

> **Ryan** and **Amy** have been married for ten years. Ryan suffers from SAD. His symptoms include feeling lethargic, sleeping way more than usual, and weight gain. He also has almost no interest in sex. Amy complains about their lack of physical closeness. Ryan spirals into a cesspool of negative thinking. He believes Amy is planning to divorce him. Ryan fills out a SAD Thought Tracker and then jots down his most troubling thought: *I know that Amy is planning on leaving me. I am a fat pig and useless in bed.*
>
> While meeting with their therapist, Ryan and Amy talk about Ryan's fears. As they talked, the therapist completed a Checking Thoughts Out Form and then had Ryan rate the results. His form is shown in Table 10-5.

Table 10-5	Ryan's Checking Thoughts Out
Questions to Check Out Thoughts	*Answers or Data I Receive*
Are you finding me less desirable?	I thought you weren't interested in me! I still want you.
Have you been considering a divorce?	Of course not, where did you get that idea?
How can we make our relationship better?	How about we take a vacation somewhere sunny and that's away from our families?
I'm feeling pretty tired at night. Could we try getting together in the daytime?	We could have a lunch date when we could be alone tomorrow!

Rating the Results:

Amy and I had a great talk. I was making up all kinds of horrors in my head. I'm really glad I checked those thoughts out. They don't hold water at all. I'm looking forward to our vacation, and my sadness has gone from about 85 to 15.

Ryan discovered that his negative thoughts were groundless. More often than not, depressed thoughts fail the test of checking them out against reality. Working with a therapist as Ryan and Amy did is only one approach for checking your thoughts out.

When you have such thoughts, try one of these strategies:

✔ **Go to the source.** Approach the person that you think harbors negative thoughts or feelings about you and ask if your assumption is correct (be sure to ask when the person has time to talk and is in a good mood).

On occasion, "going to the source" can produce negative feedback. You may hear that someone actually doesn't like you or has some negative feelings. So, you need to know that you can handle whatever you hear. If you fear that you can't handle the news, don't use this approach. On the other hand, it's often quite useful to receive such information and sometimes you can improve the relationship with that knowledge. Consult a therapist if this strategy feels too scary.

✔ **Do a survey.** Take a survey of a few close friends and ask their opinions about your negative thought. Again, make sure that you ask your friends at good times.

✔ **Act opposite.** Try "acting as if." In other words, if you feel inadequate, try acting with confidence; if you fear rejection, try approaching someone anyway. If this idea sounds too intimidating, consider looking for professional assistance.

✔ **Run a test.** Try testing out your negative predictions and track how they actually turn out. We've found that about 90 percent of the time (or more), such predictions are far more pessimistic than the actual outcomes. For example, if you decide to make a dreaded speech, be sure to write down your observations of the audience's response. You can also ask some people afterwards what they thought.

Every once in a while you may receive a negative response to one of your attempts to check out your thoughts with one of the techniques above. If that happens, take a look at some of the coping strategies in Chapters 11 and 12. If you keep putting your thoughts to the test, you may receive more positive than negative responses. If not, you probably could use some assistance from a mental health professional.

Stepping Back From Your Troubles

Have you ever heard the expression, *In your face?* This phrase refers to someone intimidating you by being too close. It's usually associated with anger, irritation, or aggression. In this case, it's your own disturbing emotions that are in your face.

In this section, we show you how to step back from your emotions a little. Doing so enables you to see things more clearly. Overly intense emotions cloud vision like a low hanging fog. Stepping away allows the fog to lift so you can gain a better perspective. Three strategies can help you get a little distance from your emotions:

✔ Putting time on your side

✔ Getting a little help from your friends

✔ Imagining the worst

You need to complete a SAD Thought Tracker form before applying these strategies. That form is seen in Chapter 9 and is also outlined in the section "Unscrambling reality scramblers" in this chapter.

Flipping the calendar ahead

One of the best ways for getting a better perspective on things is to ask yourself how you feel about some unpleasant event that's just happened at some future point in time. It's amazing how often people report feeling extremely distraught about some occurrence, but when asked how they think they'll feel in a week, a month, or a year, they typically say the current distress will no longer have much impact or meaning. Let Emma show you how it's done:

> **Emma** suffers from SAD but is having a particularly tough time this winter. She has bouts of crying and a deep, unshakeable fatigue. It's a few weeks before Christmas, and cards from her friends and family are accumulating in her mailbox. Emma can't seem to make herself send out her own cards. The whole effort involved with buying, addressing, and mailing them seems overwhelming. She scolds herself, "When they don't get my cards, people are going to hate me. I'm a lazy, uncaring, pathetic human being. I don't even deserve friends." Emma agrees with her therapist's suggestion of filling out a Thought Tracker form. She then jots down her initial thought: *I'm a horrible person for not sending out Christmas cards. My friends are going to hate me. I feel terrible.*
>
> She follows that thought with the Putting Time on Your Side Exercise as seen in Table 10-6.

Table 10-6	Emma's Putting Time on Your Side Form		
Initial Thought (From SAD Thought Tracker): I'm a horrible person for not sending out Christmas cards. My friends are going to hate me. I feel terrible.			
How I Feel Now	*How I Feel in a Week*	*How I Feel in a Month*	*How I Feel in Two Years*
I feel horribly embarrassed and ashamed.	I'll still feel pretty bad; my friends will notice they haven't received a card.	This is sort of hard to admit, but I'm guessing my friends will have pretty much forgotten about it. I probably won't feel so bad.	In two years, I can't imagine I'll even think about it. And hopefully I'll be over my recurrent SAD and more able to do such things.

Rating the Results:

I guess I can see that I'm making a pretty big deal out of a small issue. It would be nice if I manage to get myself to send out cards, but no one is going to be as upset as I've been telling myself and down the road people will totally forget about it.

Emma finds that the Putting Time on Your Side Exercise helps her step back and gain a better perspective. Now she understands that she has been getting intensely upset over issues that will not hold great meaning in the future.

 We realize that the Putting Time on Your Side Exercise sounds pretty simplistic. However, you're likely to be surprised. Most people discover that when they take current concerns and project into the future, the concerns diminish and no longer seem as serious.

Getting by with a little help

This approach gives you a way of stepping back from your problem a little and helps you gain objectivity. It involves pretending that someone else has the same problem you do. You're likely to find that you give that "someone else" much better advice than you're currently giving yourself. This technique is surprisingly powerful. You don't need a therapist to do this exercise, but you do need a bit of an imagination. First take a look at the steps involved, and then check out Figure 10-1 for the example:

1. **Complete a SAD Thought Tracker Form (see Appendix A).**

   That form is outlined in the section "Unscrambling reality scramblers" in this chapter.

2. **Record your initial thought from your SAD Thought Tracker Form.**

3. **Picture a good, trusted friend of yours sitting in a chair across from you.**

   This friend has a thought or problem similar to yours. Imagine that your friend asks you for advice. Your friend says, "What can I do about this or am I thinking clearly?"

4. **Give your friend some advice.**

   Of course you want your advice to be honest and real. At the same time, do your best to be positive and helpful. Don't sugar coat things, but find a way to help your friend see things in a better light.

5. **Rate your results.**

   Jot down what you've discovered from the exercise and whether your emotions have changed.

Okay, it may be a little weird talking to an empty chair, but we promise this technique really can work. Ricardo found that he developed SAD after moving to the United States from Mexico. His thoughts grew darker along with the reduced sunlight. He used the technique of "getting help from your friends."

Ricardo grew up in Mérida, México. He obtains a scholarship to attend college in Minneapolis, Minnesota. He becomes depressed in his first year of studies. He speaks English fluently but has trouble understanding the fast pace of lectures given by some of his professors. He also is surprised by the severity of the winter, and he finds the early darkness oppressive. When his grades come out, he receives two Bs. Ricardo had been a straight-A student in Mexico and concludes that he's a failure and should never have come to the United States to study. He visits the Student Mental Health Center and discusses his concerns with the counselor. His counselor loans him a copy of *Seasonal Affective Disorder For Dummies* (it's amazing how often those books show up!) and tells Ricardo that SAD is a common problem, especially for students who've relocated from closer to the equator. Ricardo completes a SAD Thought Tracker Form (see Appendix A). Then he adds the Getting Help From Your Friends Exercise shown in Figure 10-1.

Change Strategy: Getting Help From Your Friends

Initial Thought (From Thought Tracker Form)

I'm an idiot; I should never have come to the United States to study. I'm not smart enough. And I must be some kind of wimp for having this much trouble with the darkness and the cold.

What I would tell my friend, Roberto, if he were sitting here asking me about these issues:

Roberto, you know you're smart. For goodness sake, you were the top student in the best high school in your home town. Yes, you aren't used to getting Bs, but you only received two of them along with four As. And you struggled to understand a couple of the professors. You may be fluent in English, but it still isn't your native tongue. Give it more time and you'll understand them better. Furthermore, you're not a wimp about winter; there's something I've been reading about called SAD that's pretty common, especially among people who move from close to the equator to far Northern or Southern regions of the world. You need to lighten up and give yourself a break.

Rating the Results:

You know, I'm sort of amazed. When I was talking to my friend Roberto, everything seemed a little different. Maybe I need to start treating myself as my own best friend. My sadness and sense of hopelessness are down about 50 percent. I just need to keep working at getting a better perspective on things.

Figure 10-1:
Ricardo's Getting Help From Your Friends notes.

Ricardo found that the strategy of Getting Help From Your Friends helped straighten out his thoughts. With more realistic thinking he discovered that his moods began to lighten up. His symptoms of SAD improved gradually as he used this technique and others.

Dealing with the worst case

We work with people all the time who spend major portions of their lives in fear of various dreaded events. These folks fear future failures, disasters, or rejections. And of course their fantasy assumes that they would be totally unable to deal with these possibilities.

Living in a state of anticipated fear can ruin your life even though many of the anticipated events rarely, if ever, happen. And, believe it or not, when actually facing really tough times, these people typically cope far better than they thought they would.

Frankly, there's nothing wrong with thinking about the future from time to time. What gets people in trouble is when they wallow in their worries repeatedly and ruin the possibility of enjoying the present.

What we want you to do now is jump to the future and work through the Imagining the Worst Exercise:

1. **Complete a SAD Thought Tracker Form (see Appendix A).**

   That form is outlined in the section "Unscrambling reality scramblers" in this chapter.

2. **Fill in the Imagining the Worst Form by jotting down your initial thought from your SAD Thought Tracker Form in your notebook.**

3. **Picture your absolute worst possible fears coming true.**

   If you fear getting cancer, imagine the doctor telling you that you have an inoperable tumor. If you fear winter, imagine the coldest, darkest, winter of your life along with a deep depression.

4. **Answer the following questions:**

   • Have I ever dealt with something like this successfully before?

   • Do I know other people who've coped with something like this; if so, how did they cope with it?

- Can I turn to someone for help or support?

- Could I grow from this challenge or find meaning from it in some way?

5. **Rate your results.**

    Jot down what you've figured out about your feelings and whether your emotions have changed.

You can see how this strategy is used in the example of Sandy below. After you've seen how she does it, consider trying it yourself.

Sandy begins to worry about the coming winter as August ends. She anticipates a horrible winter season accompanied by severe depression, fatigue, weight gain, low productivity at work, losing her job, and overwhelming feelings of guilt and shame. Her worry alone begins to erode her confidence and interferes with her ability to experience enjoyment. Unfortunately, this anxiety starts to bring on the very depression she fears.

Sandy worked with a cognitive therapist the prior winter and studied new ways of thinking, which seemed to help. She recalls an exercise called "Imagining the Worst," and decides to work through it. She starts by filling out a SAD Thought Tracker Form (See Appendix A) and then writes down her initial thought followed by the Imagining the Worst Exercise in her Change Strategy. See Figure 10-2 for her example.

Sandy found that the Imagining the Worst Exercise helped her plan for possible difficulties with the upcoming winter. Doing the exercise enabled her to see that she had more options available to her than she'd realized. Sandy knew she could see her therapist again, try light therapy, and/or turn to her cousin for support. She felt more hope than despair.

Life does come with tragedy, and bad things really do happen to good people. No one goes through an entire lifetime without some sort of pain, trauma, or loss. Accepting inevitable difficulties instead of obsessively worrying about them helps you realize that you can get through troubled times. The Imagining the Worst Exercise helps you see that you can cope.

Change Strategy: Imagining the Worst

Initial Thought (From Thought Tracker Form)

Winter is coming again. I can't stand winter. I always get depressed, and I could lose my job. My blood pressure is creeping up because of my weight gain.

Have I ever dealt with something like this successfully before?

Actually, I have. Last winter I used light therapy which helped. Then in January I started going to a cognitive therapist. The work with her was very productive. I can pull out some of those techniques and strategies again.

Do I know other people who've coped with something like this; if so, how did they cope with it?

Yes, my cousin also has SAD. She used a dawn simulator. She also found an online support group that she says helped her. I haven't even tried those yet.

Can I turn to someone for help or support?

My therapist said I could always come back to see her for booster sessions if I wanted to. In fact, she said a lot of people do. It doesn't mean I didn't learn anything or "failed." And I can always turn to my cousin; she has plenty of experience in dealing with this, and we get along great.

Could I grow from this challenge or find meaning from it in some way?

I already have. I have more empathy for other people than I did before I got SAD. I realize I can do some things about my problems. When friends or co-workers have emotional struggles they come to me now.

Rating the results:

After completing this exercise, I have more hope. I know there are things I can do. First, I am going to get started with an exercise program — that should help my blood pressure and improve my mood at the same time. I feel much less hopeless now and my despair has gone from 80 to 45.

Figure 10-2:
Sandy's Imagining the Worst Exercise.

Finding Forgiveness

People who suffer from SAD often deepen their depression by focusing on mistakes, regrets, and remorse for past deeds and failings. Figuring out how to forgive yourself and others is an essential part of healing. Forgiveness is a process that takes a little time.

Forgiving yourself

If you spend a lot of time beating yourself up over past deeds, you should seek professional help or spiritual guidance. Or if you try our ideas on self-forgiveness and find it too difficult, look for assistance.

Forgiving yourself starts with acknowledging and accepting responsibility for whatever it is that you've done and now regret. Then, if possible, apologize or make amends if it involved another person. If your regret only involves yourself, apologize to yourself. Then consider these thoughts and tips:

✔ You are, after all, a fallible human. Realize that at the time of your misdeed, you were a product of history, genes, culture, and environment. You probably didn't intend to mess up. If you did, vow to do better in the future.

✔ Try to appreciate the fact that mulling over regrets and mistakes in the past only bogs you down in the present. Realize that you can't change the past. The past is over and done. Instead, concentrate on what you want to change *now*. Stay focused on the present because it's the only part of your life you can really live in. Let go of self-abuse because in a sense it's self-indulgence.

✔ Try to appreciate that when you start trying to make changes in your life for the better, you *inevitably* stumble in the darkness and slip on the ice of life. When you do, get up, dust the snow off, and move on with care. Criticizing yourself for your falls only melts your energy and motivation for moving down the path toward a brighter, sunnier life. Just as the seasons change, so can you.

Deciding to forgive others

This item can be a little tricky for some folks. Many of our clients have reported stories of horrible hurts, abuse, and life circumstances. When we bring up the topic of forgiveness, sometimes they respond with arguments. They say, "I was hurt, I didn't deserve what happened," or "I can't possibly ever forgive after what happened to me." And why should they forgive people who've wronged them?

Turns out there are good reasons. Studies have shown the obvious — holding onto anger, and resentment leads to angry and resentful people. If you have these emotions, you can't truly be happy and satisfied at the same time.

Forgiveness doesn't mean actually declaring the grievous acts to have been okay and acceptable. Nor does forgiving discount the importance of what's happened to you in the past. Rather, forgiveness involves letting go. Letting go of negative emotions opens the door to the possibility of serenity and happiness.

Steps to forgiveness include the following:

- ✔ **Recall the offense or wrong that happened to you.** Be as impartial and objective as you can when you reflect. Step back a little from the event by imagining that you're watching it happen on a television screen.

- ✔ **Try to view the offense from the other person's perspective.** This step may feel a little difficult, especially if the wrong was particularly harsh and hurtful. However, try to get any amount of understanding of that person's view that you can.

- ✔ **Think as yourself as a survivor or a coper rather than as a victim.** In other words, develop an image of yourself as strong and empowered, not weak and helpless.

- ✔ **Forgive.** Forgiveness means that you *let go* of what's happened to you as well as the rage and resentment you may feel. In a sense, you give yourself back the life you had before the event occurred. You don't actually have to declare that the offender was "right" or "justified."

Aaron's story below illustrates the forgiveness process. Aaron finds forgiveness challenging, but worth the effort.

> **Aaron** suffered from bouts of SAD for many years. He eventually read about light therapy, which worked very well for him for four years in a row. However, six months ago Aaron was mugged while walking home from work. His anger turned to depression as fall was ending. Lights didn't help Aaron at all this time.

Aaron went to a pastoral counselor. The counselor worked with him on how to forgive. Although he found it difficult at first, Aaron eventually worked through the steps to forgiveness:

- ✔ **Recall the offense or wrong that happened to you.** Aaron talked about the mugging and eventually was able to picture the scene in his mind with a measure of objectivity like he was making a science report.

- ✔ **Try to view the offense from the other person's perspective.** Aaron realized that the mugger probably had a very difficult life, possibly filled with abuse or other traumas. This fact certainly didn't make the event "right" or "justifiable," but it helped him let go a little.

✔ **Think as yourself as a survivor or a coper rather than as a victim.** Aaron found this step especially helpful. He realized he had been viewing himself as a helpless victim. He replaced that image with one of a strong, coper.

✔ **Forgive.** The counselor told Aaron he didn't exactly have to send the mugger a gift or note saying that "all is okay." However, by forgiving, he gives himself a greater gift. He makes the decision to let go of the anger and resentment.

Like Aaron, when you forgive, you take away the power of the offender over your life. Letting go of anger, rage, and resentment allows you to regain control of your emotions and your life.

Chapter 11

Soothing the Storms Within

*E*veryone experiences bursts of bad feelings from time to time. You may encounter events that are pleasant and others that leave you feeling upset and distraught.

Think about how you felt the last time you had a flat tire, your roof leaked, someone criticized you at work, or someone you cared about left you. But don't spend too much time dwelling on such events — we don't want to set off a rotten mood!

Why are we asking you to briefly contemplate life's many lamentable yet inevitable incidents? Because people who suffer from seasonal affective disorder (SAD) commonly feel unable to cope with these unavoidable bad times. When they detect anxiety, anger, distress, and upset erupting, they can feel overwhelmed and unable to function. These reactions then lead to deeper depression.

In this chapter, you discover how to see that feelings are simply feelings. In other words, if you accept emotions as simply temporary responses to circumstances, they typically don't seem as overwhelming. Then we describe two quick skills — breathing and relaxation — both of which can help you defuse emotional eruptions, sometimes before they even start. We also provide a couple of distraction techniques that allow emotions to settle down through refocusing your attention on other activities. Next we discuss an especially intriguing way to deal with upsetting emotions by *triggering* or eliciting more pleasant feelings. The chapter concludes with a brief discussion on how to use flash cards as self-reminders when times get dicey.

Reinterpreting Feelings

When you find yourself in a particularly anguished state of mind, thinking about anything other than the terrible thoughts and feelings you're experiencing becomes difficult. Everyone gets mired in a bog of misery here and there. It's part of being human.

For example, we teach psychology graduate students who for the most part are highly intelligent and reasonably well-balanced folks from an emotional standpoint. However, when they receive negative feedback on their academic performance, they commonly wallow in self-loathing and feelings of despair, at least for a while. They sometimes compound the problem by berating themselves for having such feelings; after all, they're training to be mental health professionals who "shouldn't" feel this way.

However, disturbing emotional storms linger, intensify, and remain far longer when you tell yourself that they're terrible, awful, and something that you simply *must* not have. But there's an alternative way of looking at sad or distressing feelings.

 Stop evaluating and judging the distress and remind yourself that feelings are nothing more than feelings, whether they feel good or bad. And all feelings eventually dissipate; with enough time, even emotional hurricanes move on. When emotions threaten to flood your mind and soul with darkness, try repeating this phrase to yourself over and over again: *Feelings are just feelings. All feelings will pass. In the meantime, I can simply observe them and accept their presence in my life for the moment.* You may also find it useful to read Chapter 18 for more info on acceptance.

Relying on Relaxation

Some people don't know how to regulate their emotional states. And most of these individuals had parents who modeled emotional dyscontrol (the inability to control one's feelings). When you spend much of your childhood observing people who exhibit tempers, distress, and upset without also demonstrating healthy resolutions to these outbursts, you may experience difficulty with managing your own emotions. You never figured out how, so we can help.

 Relaxation is something that you can't *force* to occur. Instead, you allow it to come over you slowly. The harder you try to *make* yourself relax, the less successful you'll be. Give the process time. Try out some relaxation tapes available in bookstores and on the Internet if you need extra help getting to the point of relaxation.

Relaxation is a skill. Like any skill, it takes time to master. Be sure to practice relaxation as close to everyday as you can. It doesn't have to take much time; regularity is more important than the total amount of time you devote to it.

Two related skills can help you manage through periodic emotional tsunamis when they strike. No skills allow you to completely eliminate or control all distressing feelings. The skills in this section help prevent some of these events or reduce their intensity when they do occur. These skills are breathing and progressive muscle relaxation.

Using your breathing to cope

Okay, you already know how to breathe. If you didn't, you wouldn't have made it this far in life, right? With that said, you probably breathed the "right way" as an infant and have done it wrong pretty much ever since.

As an infant the baby's stomach rises and falls with each and every breath as it goes in and out. Yet most adults breathe by holding their stomachs in and using their chests to move the air in and out. (This is probably in part from parents telling their kids to hold their stomachs in, so chest breathing becomes an ingrained habit.)

People also breathe too quickly — especially in response to stress, which often feels like the right thing to do, but it isn't. Excessive rapid breathing can cause an excess of oxygen and a state called *hyperventilation*. Hyperventilation can cause jitteriness, rapid pulse, blurred vision, confusion, feelings of panic, and even loss of consciousness. As you can imagine, these symptoms don't exactly help you feel better when emotional distress occurs.

So to help you combat your distress, there's a better way to breathe. Try practicing the following steps five minutes a day for two weeks before you try and apply it to an attack of emotional upset. That way, you understand the technique well and are better able to use it under duress.

This exercise is called *abdominal breathing,* and with it you figure out how to breathe with your diaphragm instead of your chest, which helps you relax better. Follow these steps:

1. **Find a spot to lie down or find a large chair that you can really stretch out in.**

   Notice the tension in your body and rate it on a 10-point scale with 1 representing little or no tension and 10 indicating the maximal imaginable amount of tension.

2. **Place one hand on your stomach and take in a very slow, deep breath through your nose while attempting to fill up the lower part of your lungs first.**

   It's easy to tell if you're doing this part correctly because your hand rises slightly as you breathe in. Pause and hold that breath for a few seconds.

3. **Slowly exhale, allowing the bottom portion of your lungs to exhale first and see that your hand goes down as you do.**

   As you exhale, imagine that your body is like a balloon filled with air that's slowly deflating. Take a brief pause once more.

4. **Inhale slowly and deeply while filling the lower part of your lungs first.**

   Sometimes it helps to inhale to a slow count of four. Make sure that your hand rises as you inhale. Keep your chest movement to a minimum — it should rise only slightly.

5. **Pause and slowly exhale again.**

   Try to exhale to a slow count of six. You may start with a count of four if you need to, but a count of six becomes easier with practice.

6. **Continue to breathe in this manner for about five minutes.**

   While you do, focus only on your breathing. If unpleasant thoughts start to intrude, just notice them and refocus on your breathing when you can.

7. **Notice what tension remains in your body and rate it on the same scale of 1 to 10 as before.**

   Just five minutes a day and you're likely to find that abdominal breathing starts reducing your stress levels and helps you take the edge off emotional distress when it strikes. The more you practice abdominal breathing, the lower your tension ratings are likely to be.

You're busy, but everyone can find five minutes a day for this useful exercise. If you don't think so, it's probably just a sign of your tense mind trying to convince you that nothing can change for the better. But it can.

Putting your muscles to work

Tension in the mind usually leads to excessive tension in your body's muscles. And tight muscles increase the feelings of tension in the mind. It's a vicious cycle. Progressive muscle relaxation can stop the tension cycle.

Progressive muscle relaxation was developed by Dr. Edmund Jacobsen (a physician living in Chicago) just prior to the dawn of World War II. Progressive muscle relaxation became widely used and has since been found to provide relief for a wide range of ailments:

✔ Chronic pain

✔ Insomnia

✔ Headaches

✔ Anxiety

✔ Emotional distress

Other studies have even found that progressive muscle relaxation may slightly improve the functioning of your immune system. This technique is highly useful.

Many variations of progressive muscle relaxation have been developed. You can do an Internet search for *progressive muscle relaxation* and find dozens of sites with specific instructions for each variation or you can find the instructions in a wide range of books. We present you a *highly abbreviated* form of progressive muscle relaxation. If you find that this quick strategy doesn't work for you, try one of the longer versions posted on the Internet or in *Overcoming Anxiety For Dummies* (Wiley) — a book we happened to write, too.

Here's how it works:

1. **Find a comfortable place to lie down or stretch out.**

   Minimize distractions — turn off phones, pull down the shades, and so on. Some sounds may break through from the outside, but just return to your relaxation after you hear them.

2. **Notice whatever tension you have in your body and rate it on a scale of 1 (almost none) to 10 (extreme).**

3. **Take a slow deep breath, hold it a few moments, and slowly exhale.**

   Ideally, you can use the abdominal breathing technique in the earlier section "Using your breathing to cope." Repeat this breath three or four times.

4. **Tighten your hands, arms, shoulders, and upper back.**

   Bring your shoulders up and imagine yourself like a turtle trying to get into its shell. Hold the tension for a few seconds and notice it. Don't tighten so much that you cause pain or discomfort.

5. **Then all at once, let go of the tension and let your hands, arms, and shoulders drop, allowing relaxation to slowly flow in as the tension flows out.**

   Spend a few moments allowing that process to take place.

6. **Keep your hands, arms, shoulders, and back as relaxed as you can and tighten up the muscles in your face, head, and neck.**

   Notice the tension and hold it for a few seconds. Don't allow the tension to create discomfort and then let go of the tension all at once and allow relaxation to slowly come in and take its place.

7. **Tighten the muscles in your stomach and chest while keeping the other muscle groups as relaxed as possible.**

   Hold that tension a few moments. Then let it go. Allow feelings of relaxation to slowly take the place of the tension as it drains away.

8. **Contract the muscles in the lower part of your body, including your buttocks, thighs, calves, and feet.**

   Hold the tension a few moments and then let it go all at once. Notice the tension flowing out and relaxation coming in to take its place.

9. **Take a short tour through your body in your mind and notice if there are any remaining areas of tension.**

   If tension remains, take a few moments to allow the relaxed areas around them come in and replace the tension. Tighten specific areas for a few moments and then let it go while giving relaxation a second chance to come in place of the tension.

10. **Spend a few minutes noticing the way your body feels while you also take a few slow, deep breaths.**

    Hold each breath a few seconds and let it go slowly. Let relaxation spread and notice any feelings of warmth, gentle sinking, or floating.

11. **Rate the tension in your body on a 1- to 10-point scale and see if you succeeded at reducing the tension in your body.**

Although somewhat unusual, sometimes people actually feel some discomfort or distress when trying relaxation. There's a simple solution — just stop if you feel this way. If it keeps happening, seek professional help if you really want to continue with relaxation. Furthermore, please avoid tightening any part of the body that's injured or tends to act up on you — like your lower back.

Make a tape recording of this procedure, talking through the steps and then listening to the recording as you do the exercise. Be sure you speak very slowly and in a calm, even tone of voice.

Checking Out Your Options for Distractions

You can approach alleviating emotional turmoil by using distractions — various ways of focusing your mind on things that can help you stop the constant pounding thoughts telling you how terrible things are and why you should and do feel horrible. Check out ways to stop the distress in following sections.

Counting

Counting can refocus your thoughts and get you back on track. Try this simple exercise:

1. **Sit or lie down in a comfortable position.**
2. **Start counting backwards from 100 and slowly count down to zero.**

   If you lose your place, start over. Notice each number and visualize it in your mind. It's difficult to focus on distressing thoughts and feelings while you're concentrating on counting and actually seeing the numbers in your head.

Doing puzzles

Putting your mind to the grind and challenging your smarts can help you focus your positive energy. Try a puzzle or two. Some people like jigsaw puzzles; others love crossword puzzles. The options in this area are endless.

Try out the hot Japanese mind/numbers game known as Sudoku. In fact, you can even get *Sudoku For Dummies* by Andrew Heron and Edmund James (Wiley) in three different volumes. This puzzle craze is rather addictive and can conceivably keep your mind sharper as you age.

Reading a good book

Reading uses a lot more brain power than watching television, and it does a much better job of distracting you from upsetting thoughts and feelings. Have a few highly engaging novels out and ready to read. These books don't need to be literary masterpieces, just something that engages your mind.

Enjoying media

No doubt you have some music that you enjoy. Pick some selections that you enjoy when you're in a good mood and have these choices handy to pop in the CD player when you aren't feeling as great. Make sure your choices have an upbeat quality to them.

Are you a movie buff? Do you prefer to curl up with a psychological thriller or belly laugh at a comical flick? If you have a movie collection, set aside a few comedies or some of your favorite movies. Then when you're feeling stressed, pull one of these selections out and tune in so you can tune out.

Changing your temperature

Sudden temperature changes can switch on better feelings. You can try this tactic through two different methods.

The first method probably won't surprise you — take a really hot, long bath or soak in a hot tub. Warm water helps muscles relax. That's the idea behind hot tubs and saunas.

The second strategy is going to sound well, weird. When your emotions feel overheated, try the following:

1. **Fill a bowl or a sink with ice water.**

   That's right — water and ice cubes.

2. **Take a deep breath and plunge your face into the water.**

3. **Hold your face in the water as long as you can and then come up for air.**

4. **Repeat Steps 2 and 3 once or twice.**

   You're very likely to forget what's troubling you. By the way, we wouldn't suggest something to you that we haven't tried ourselves — it's not nearly as awful as it may sound! An alternative distraction is to use an ice bag and put it on your face or arm.

Slap a smile on your face

When all else fails, smile — a slight smile, like a Mona Lisa smile. You don't have to smile around other people, but it's a good idea because when you do, others usually smile back. You may be surprised by how much smiling can improve your mood.

Studies have actually found that pulling your facial muscles into a slight smile helps you feel better. Why? Probably because of the association that's been made so many times in your life between smiling and feeling good. Thus, even if you don't feel good currently, smiling can help bring the more positive feelings on.

Using Flash Cards to Cope

Remember flash cards from elementary school that your teacher used to help you master those multiplication tables? This technique uses a similar approach for figuring out how to cope! Having a plan in hand goes a long way toward giving you a sense of control when emotions swell up.

Here's how the flash cards work:

1. **Get a 3-x-5-inch or 4-x-6-inch index card.**
2. **At the top of the card write** *My Coping Plan.*
3. **List four or five strategies that you want to remember to do whenever dark emotions threaten to erupt.**

   Ideally, you've tried out all these strategies in the past and found them to work. This card should fit in your pocket, briefcase, or purse. The reason it helps is that when powerful emotions take hold, people's memories typically turn off. You're likely to benefit from a reminder.

Check out this example:

> **Olivia,** a child psychotherapist, enjoys her work with children and families. She's well known in town and considered an expert in her field. She takes on difficult cases but is clear with her clients that she doesn't wish to get involved in child custody cases. These cases often become centered on the divorcing parents' wish to get back at each other and have little to do with what is best for the child.
>
> Olivia is stunned and startled when a disheveled young man opens the door to her office without knocking. He crosses the room quickly and says, "Olivia," and hands her some papers. She's mad when she realizes she was tricked into taking a subpoena. She glances at the name and isn't surprised to see that it's a demand to testify in a trial regarding the divorced parents of a child she's recently seen. Her anger grows when she starts thinking about all the clients who she has to cancel, the distance of traveling to the courtroom, and the well-known adversarial climate of the courtroom. So Olivia, having previously prepared a coping plan for herself, pulls out her card and starts going through the list until she feels her emotions calming down.
>
> Since she's at her office, she isn't going to do #4 (putting her face in ice water) because it would ruin her makeup. But she does decide to try abdominal breathing, followed by reminding herself repeatedly that all such intense upsets do pass with a little time. She finds herself feeling a little better within five minutes. Fifteen minutes later she's almost back to her usual self. In the past, events like this kept her in a bad mood most of the day.

Check out Figure 11-1 for a picture of what Olivia's index card looks like and how to construct your own.

My Coping Plan _____

1. I will try abdominal breathing for five minutes.

2. I will work on a puzzle for at least five minutes.

3. I will count very slowly from 1 to 100.

4. I will try the face in ice water trick. It really helps even though it always sounds awful to me so I have to remind myself that it really helps.

5. I will remind myself that I have never had an emotional eruption last more than a day or so and that they usually lessen much sooner than that. So, I'll tell myself, "This too shall pass" over and over and over.

Figure 11-1:
Olivia's
coping plan.

When you design your card, feel free to use any strategy that works for you. It doesn't have to be on our list! Make sure that at least one technique can be done in public places — such as counting backward or a simplified breathing strategy (you don't have to be stretched out on a large chair).

Chapter 12

Handling SAD Stress

Stress is a combination of your emotional, physical, and mental responses to life. Both good things and bad things can be stressors. But generally, most folks view stress as a normal reaction to having too much to do, feeling overwhelmed, sitting in traffic, answering a message from your boss, or even reading the daily newspaper. Stress follows you most days, like your shadow. As long as you're alert and alive, you experience stress. But, what does stress have to do with seasonal affective disorder (SAD)?

Too much stress seems to go hand in hand with depression. If you already suffer from SAD, stress can make your symptoms worse. In this chapter, we tell you about the connection of stress to depression. Then we give you tips on letting go of inessentials, figuring out daily goals, and getting help when you need it. Then we give you some hints about stress-free thinking.

Connecting Depression and Stress

For most people, having a flat tire and spilling coffee on themselves in the same day is annoying but, ultimately, no big deal. They shake these events off and move on. Not so for a SAD sufferer; a day like could feel like the end of the world. The impact of negative stress seems magnified through the lens of SAD or depression.

For someone prone to SAD, a day filled with a series of mishaps can actually trigger a lasting depressive episode. Someone not prone to SAD or depression may feel "depressed" from having to deal with a full day of negative stressors but can manage to work through each event and, again, move on after a short time.

So, the relationship between depression and stress runs two ways. When you're depressed, even the small stuff seems pretty big. And when you have too much stress, it's easy to become depressed. So, it's another one of those chicken and egg deals — no one really knows which one comes first.

However, science has looked at stressful events that seem linked to depression. If you have one or more of the following stressors, you may be at risk for becoming depressed, or if you're already depressed, your symptoms could worsen. You can find various lists of what are typically considered major stressors on the Internet and in professional journals. The following list gives you a flavor of what are considered serious stressors:

- A long, daily commute in heavy traffic
- Being a victim of a crime or terrorist attack
- Being diagnosed with a serious and/or chronic illness
- Being transferred to a new city
- Buying or building a new home
- Family violence or conflict
- Having a baby
- Loss of a relationship from breakup, death, or distance
- Serious financial stress
- Taking care of a handicapped or sick family member

You may notice that a couple of the items above could be considered good things — such as having a baby or buying or building a new home. However, such undertakings require many decisions, considerable time, large financial implications, and various changes in lifestyle. Even if the ultimate result is good, stress goes along for the ride.

Severe stress may change the chemistry of your body by increasing cortisol and adrenaline, which can contribute to depression. Fact is, stress can kill you if you don't figure out how to manage it. Stress-related illnesses include the following:

- Cardiac problems, such as high blood pressure
- Chronic pain

> ✔ Gastrointestinal problems, such as irritable bowel syndrome (IBS)
>
> ✔ Insomnia

Researchers have even discovered that people under long-term stress appear to experience genetic changes that are usually associated with aging. In fact, the saying that someone "aged overnight," is related to real changes at the molecular level of the body that occurs from acute stress.

This chapter focuses on chronic, long-term stressors that slowly wear you down. For ideas on how to deal with short-term stressors and the accompanying emotional reactions to them, see Chapter 11.

Resetting Your Priorities

So, how do you start knocking stress out of your life? One of the best ways of reducing chronic stress is to *reprioritize* your life. If you're like most people, you never deal with what you value and feel is truly important. Why? Because you probably haven't taken the time to think about and decide what kind of life you want to live.

Do you ever say to yourself that you're too busy? Does it seem that by the time you work, shop for groceries, pay the bills, cook, clean up, and check your e-mail that the day is gone? How do the days, weeks, months, and years fly by so quickly? What do these questions have to do with reprioritizing your life?

Well, in order to reprioritize you have to know what's happening with your life right now. This task is more difficult when you're down as may be the case during a cold winter. However, you can still set goals so you fill your days with more of what you want and less of what's unimportant. Finally, you carry out your goals and start living the life you want to live.

You start the process by taking some time to keep a log of what you did last week. Check out Table 12-1 for an example. You might say to yourself, *I don't have time to do one more thing.* You don't have to make this entry an essay, just a few quick notes. Here's an example to get you started:

> **David,** a busy attorney, suffered from SAD for five winters in a row. However, last year he used light therapy (see Chapter 5) and cognitive behavior therapy (see Chapters 9 and 10) and successfully conquered his SAD. However, his psychologist tells him that he can reduce his risks of a recurrence of SAD if he deals with his chronic stress and reprioritizes his life.

Table 12-1	David's Activity Log
Day of the Week	**Day's Activities**
Monday	Today I had my usual hour commute to work. Attended a long meeting in the morning, had a luncheon with some attorneys. Stopped at the grocery store; it was cold and dark, and I slipped on the ice in the parking lot. I got home after 6:30 p.m. My wife and I ate a light dinner and then I went into the office and checked e-mail. It was nine o'clock when I noticed the time. Went in and watched TV until bed.
Tuesday	Same day as yesterday. But I didn't stop at the grocery store. I did go to the post office to send off a package during my lunch hour. Read my e-mail and watched TV again.
Wednesday	So, I'm getting the point. I really did the same thing today. I am bored at work and really pretty bored with what I do in the evenings. It feels even worse when it gets dark this early.
Thursday	Ditto. Same old, same old.
Friday	Hooray it's the weekend. My wife and I went to the neighborhood brewery after work and had pizza and a couple of beers. We were both tired and came home and went to bed watching the news channel.
Saturday	Went grocery shopping. What a mad house. Then we went to the mall. Needed some new towels for the guest room. I had planned to get a jog in today but by the time we got home from the mall I didn't feel like it. We rented a movie and chilled out.
Sunday	Got up and sat around drinking coffee and reading the paper. Did a little e-mail and then had to go over to my mother-in-law's house for a visit. I did get in a short jog with the dog this afternoon. Even though it was really cold, I felt a little rejuvenated. Watched TV and went to bed early.

David's log for the week in Table 12-1 gives him insight into how he spends his time. He begins to beat himself up for leading such a dull life. He believes that he's letting life slip away watching TV, working at an unfulfilling job, and doing mundane chores.

But there's a second step after listing your week's activities. Dream a bit and think about what you want to accomplish. Think about your career, your family, your community, your finances, your body, and your mind. How do you want to live your life? Get out some paper and write down your ideas. Then pick one or two of your ideas as goals that you want to focus on. Follow these steps:

1. **Make your goals specific, measurable, and obtainable.**

   How long will it take you to reach your goal? Be sure that you're able to tell when you've accomplished your goal.

2. **Break your goals down into small steps.**

   Don't say you want to write the world's greatest novel next week. Try coming up with a title or an idea. In other words, the smaller the steps, the better.

3. **Try to be realistic yet feel free to dream (don't promise world peace, unless you're the president of a big country; even then . . .).**

4. **Review and celebrate success.**

   When you've reached your goal, decide if you need a new goal or want to expand on the current one. Give yourself a pat on the back for making a positive change in your life.

Table 12-2 is a sample of David's goals. Notice the goals don't have to be anything earth shaking. You simply need to come up with ideas for giving your life a little more focus on the things that you value.

Table 12-2	**David's Goal Chart**
Goal	*Possible Action Steps*
I want to have more time to hike, jog, and be active. I know that being outside can help my SAD.	I'll talk to my boss about flexing my time. I could save four hours a week in traffic if I worked four ten-hour days. Then I can have a day during the week to hike, jog, or take care of errands when it's less busy.
	There's a grocery store in town that delivers groceries that you order online. Because I usually sit in front of my computer in the evening, my wife and I can come up with a list and hike on Saturday's instead of grocery shopping.

(continued)

Table 12-2 *(continued)*

Goal	Possible Action Steps
	I can walk to the train station each morning and catch the Metro express to work. That way I get more walking into my life, and I can actually do a little work on the ride. All I have to do is be sure to dress warmly enough on the really cold days.
I want to contribute to my community.	There's a three-year waiting list for Big Brothers in my county. Volunteering only takes about an hour a week. I can do this opportunity, especially since I've started on flex time at work.
	Our neighborhood is always looking for volunteers. I've always wanted to participate more actively. I can start by organizing a neighborhood cleanup — more exercise for me and a cleaner neighborhood to boot. Now that's a deal.
	I can volunteer to be on the Fourth of July committee for our town's celebration. That sounds like fun. That way, I can look forward to the summer even though it's a little dreary out there now.

David starts the ball rolling. He asks his boss about flex time and is told the request will be considered, but not for another month or two. He lets himself feel good about what he's done so far. In addition, he notices that he's lost a few pounds (instead of his usual eight-pound winter weight gain) because of the increased walking to the train station each day and the up tick in his hiking. His mood starts improving.

David's second goal and possible action steps are "doable." David enjoys meeting new neighbors and connecting with others. He becomes a Big Brother and feels a greater sense of purpose and meaning. He no longer resents the aimlessness of his life. He takes the time every six months or so to design a new goal for himself.

It's never a good idea to come up with unrealistic grand schemes. You may decide to make your goals larger at some point, but start with relatively achievable ones in the beginning. You don't have to carry out all of your action steps and some may prove "undoable." That's okay; just make a list and do the ones you can.

Cleaning Out the Junk in Your Life

Part of helping you deal with your SAD is de-stressing your life. When you get organized, you can become more efficient and start spending your time more the way you want to and less on endless searches for things. Clutter and disorganization create stress.

Getting organized also includes *getting rid of stuff* — lots and lots of stuff. And sometimes letting go is hard to do. Whether it's that blue shirt that you like but haven't worn in two years, or those replaced plumbing parts you thought you might use someday — there always seems to be a reason for keeping things. But as stuff accumulates and clutter grows, it becomes harder and harder to find the really useful things, and your stress rises. Letting go and getting rid of what you don't need helps lighten your stress in the long run.

You don't have to do everything at once. When stuff has accumulated over years, it takes awhile to get fully organized. Just do what you can. For example, toss one garbage bag full of junk each weekend or spend 30 minutes two nights a week on the project. Over six months, you can clear out an astounding amount of clutter.

Just in case we've convinced you it may be worthwhile to toss out and organize what's left, here are a few tips to get started:

✔ **Scour your closet.** If you haven't worn something in over a year, out it goes! If you want to make an exception for one, single item, okay. But otherwise, toss! You may be surprised how difficult this purging feels, but when you're done, you'll feel better. At the same time, appreciate that a needy person can benefit if you take the used clothes to charity.

✔ **Clean out your bathroom.** How many extra travel bottles of shampoo, lotions, and hairspray do you need? If you have a half or quarter bottle of one lotion, dump it into another half-full one. De-clutter by putting similar items together. Consider buying a few inexpensive plastic tubs or shelves that fit in your cupboards.

✔ **Purge those old books.** How many old novels take up space on your bookshelves? Go through your books and eliminate the ones you know you're never going to read again. Donate them to your public library — it usually has a way of making use of them. You could also sell them in a garage sale, at a used bookstore, or even on the Internet.

✔ **Clean out your garage.** Aaaack — we can hear your screams from here. Pick a nice day; pull everything out and toss (donate) the items you aren't likely to need. Organize, put up a pegboard, add a few shelves, whatever you need to do. Get a tall, narrow garbage can to hold all your snow shovels and rakes. Hang items on the wall or from the ceiling. You can do this! If it seems overwhelming, consider doing one half or one corner at a time. But be sure to schedule the time in and do it.

✔ **Organize your bills, taxes, and papers.** Make files for your bills and papers. Make files for your taxes. After you have files, take 30 seconds to put each item away. Tax records need to be kept for a long time, but you can store them in a storage shed. Supportive documents for your personal taxes or business need to be kept for three years and six years, respectively. But if you're not sure, consult a tax professional. And you can consult the Internet for how long experts recommend keeping other types of receipts.

When tossing financial records of any type, be sure to buy a personal shredder and grind them up before you throw them. Identity theft is on the rise, and you don't want to become the next victim.

✔ **Clean out your drawers.** Most kitchens and bedrooms are filled with drawers and various nooks and crannies stuffed with junk. Again, unless you figure the odds are 50 percent or greater that you'll need an item in the next year or so, donate it!

✔ **Make a rule when you buy something new, toss at least one item out.** Trust us; this rule makes a difference over time.

Taking our own advice

We modestly admit to being pretty good psychologists. Furthermore, we can write a darn decent book (if we do say so ourselves) when we set our minds to it. And setting our minds to a task happens with surprising frequency. When we write books, we spend considerable time researching. We have fun exploring the Internet where you can obtain almost every article ever written from journals, newspapers, and magazines. And that's pretty much what we do.

After we print those articles, we arrange them in neat geological layers on our desks. Well, not so neat. And that's not to mention the piles on our credenza; oh, and then there's the banquet tables set up in our office. And of course sometimes we actually go to our day jobs and miss a few days of writing. So when we return to writing, we have pretty much forgotten which articles are where, so we start digging through them again.

Then, feeling hopeless, we go back to the Internet and rediscover some of the same articles that lie buried deeply in some obscure pile. Nevertheless, we reprint it, only to start a new pile. Does this process sound a little inefficient to you?

Well, it is! So, we've made a decision while writing this chapter. After *this* book is finished, we're going to organize our office. We're even considering a broader project and are planning to set aside two weeks to see what we can accomplish. We feel better just thinking about getting organized!

Dematerializing

By dematerializing we don't mean to vanish into thin air like people did in the transporter on the Starship Enterprise. Instead, start realizing that, for most people, money takes a lot of time and energy to earn. When you spend it frivolously, you create more stress on yourself to earn more. Obviously, there's no single answer as to what constitutes *frivolous*. However, you can probably start saving a lot of dough if you redefine *frivolous* for yourself.

Billions of dollars are spent on advertising designed to convince you that you absolutely must have the latest car, the most fashionable clothes, the fastest computer, the smallest cell phone in the world, and the latest in bathroom redesign. And the ads try to tell you that true happiness can't be found without all these things. But ask yourself a question. On a scale of 1 to 10, how much did the last car you bought or the clothes hanging in your closet really increase your overall happiness? Or, think of it another way; how quickly did buyer's remorse set in after your last significant purchase?

When you start throwing things out (see preceding section "Cleaning Out the Junk in Your Life"), ask yourself how much it all cost and to what extent it really improved your life satisfaction. Make a decision to stop buying all that junk. You can work less and have more time for what really matters. Leave more money in your bank account and ask yourself a few questions that can help you make better purchasing decisions in the future:

- ✔ **Do you really need it or just want it?** Ask yourself this question before making any purchase and be sure to answer honestly. You may surprise yourself at how much you *want* to buy but what you don't really *need* when you stop to think about it.

- ✔ **Do you need as much as you're buying or could you use less?** The discount warehouse clubs are great, but often require that large quantities of foods and other items be purchased. Soup may be a few cents cheaper per can when bought by the case, but will you really use it all? Not everything is a bargain in bulk!

- ✔ **Do you need it now or could it wait?** Early adopters are those people who run out and buy the newest gizmo as soon as it hits the market. They also pay the highest prices. Waiting can pay off because prices fall, or items go on sale. If you don't truly need it now, wait.

- ✔ **Do you need it new or is used okay?** Secondhand clothing shops abound and are full of wonderful "gently worn" items that look like new but cost only a fraction of the original price. And a used book reads just as well as a new one!

Outsourcing Your Chores

Seeking out help costs money, and if you read the preceding section on dematerializing your life, which suggests looking for ways to stop spending frivolously, you may think we're contradicting ourselves. Not really. We do suggest you hire such help only after careful consideration. Reasons that support seeking such help can include the following:

- ✔ **You've tried many times without success.** If in spite of your best intentions, you've been utterly unable to get yourself organized, you may need some help. This help is most likely a one-time investment instead of an ongoing cost.

- ✔ **You have money but not time.** If you earn a good income that allows you to hire outside help that frees up your time, then it's a good investment. On the other hand, it doesn't make a lot of sense to hire help and then take on a second job to cover the additional cost.

- ✔ **You lack the needed expertise.** We've tried to repair our sprinkler system in the past and found it turns into a full-day project. We stare at piles of plastic and rubber parts in disorder and disarray. Then we go to our local hardware store and painstakingly search the aisles. We usually buy gobs of extra parts because it's sort of hard to tell which ones actually do the job. Then we spend the afternoon trying to get it all to work. After we get drenched from our repair attempts, we end up calling the experts who come out and fix the problem in 15 minutes. Sometimes, it's worth it to make the call instead of trying to fix something you know nothing about.

If any of the above reasons are staring you in the face and if you're a little overwhelmed with getting some chores done around the house, professional organizers exist who come to your home and hold your hand through the entire job. They save you money in the long run by getting your life back on the track to efficiency and greater productivity. Just like big companies that outsource jobs, you can outsource some of your routine tasks to save you loads of time.

Before you hire someone to organize your home and/or office, you should check that person out. Certain vulnerabilities can exist in letting someone else go through your stuff with you, so you need to be completely comfortable with the person you choose. Check with the Better Business Bureau, friends, references provided by the organizer, and even consumer rating companies on the Internet, such as www.angieslist.com to find the person right for you and your needs.

Help is available for other areas of your life as well. Here are a few of the possibilities:

✔ **Bookkeeping or financial planning:** Some people hate even thinking about money issues. They hate paying bills or making investment decisions. Help is available. When hiring a financial advisor, make sure he's not more motivated by generating commissions than in looking out for your best interests.

✔ **Cleaning:** Some people simply hate to clean. If that's you, consider getting a maid. Services include spring or winter cleaning; you don't have to hire them year-round. If you're suffering from SAD, consider hiring such a service as a way of getting you through the winter. On the other hand, you may consider combining some of your exercise goals with cleaning your own house — just do it aerobically and you can kill two birds with one stone.

✔ **Gardening and household maintenance:** If these tasks simply aren't your cup of tea, consider hiring help for them. Again, check out anyone you hire for work around your house.

✔ **Meal preparation:** This idea may be one you choose to do only in the winter, when your energy reserves are lower, but your choices abound. At the high end of this category are personal chefs. They aren't as expensive as they sound, and some even deliver a week's worth of meals to your home.

Somewhat less expensive services include ones where you go to the location once a month, pick out a menu, make a number of meals with pre-measured ingredients and helpful instructions, bag the meals, and freeze them.

Finding More Ways to Knock Out Stress

Leave no stone unturned in your quest to reduce stress in your life, and so this section offers a few more ideas for reducing stress. Give them a try because as you reduce stress you're likely to feel less effects of your SAD and happier to boot.

Saying no more often

Why is it so hard for people to say no? People want to be nice when they can. So it's not surprising when someone asks you to do something, that you find yourself saying yes. But sometimes you find yourself resenting your decision later. If that's the case, you probably need to figure out how to say no.

And indeed sometimes people might get upset with you when you start saying no and setting limits. But you have to realize that you can only do what you can do. And feeling stressed and resentful is truly inflicting harm on yourself.

Try some good ways to say no that don't have to offend anyone. Here are a few:

- ✔ I'd love to, but my schedule is just too full.
- ✔ That just won't work for me.
- ✔ I wish I could, but I can't take more on right now.
- ✔ Something just doesn't feel right about that to me. I'm afraid I just have to say no.
- ✔ No thanks.
- ✔ I'm trying to avoid new projects and responsibilities right now.
- ✔ Sorry; I have other commitments that are tying me up.
- ✔ I'd like to, but I have to put my focus on my family.
- ✔ That sounds interesting, but my agenda is too full.
- ✔ I'd like to, but I have some priorities that need to be addressed first.
- ✔ I don't think that sounds like something I'd enjoy.
- ✔ I'm sorry; I think I'm going to pass on that one.

Write the above ways to say no out on a 3-x-5-inch index card or make a note in your daily planner or your PDA. Practice saying them over and over again. Remind yourself that you have an absolute right to say no. You can't be all things to all people all the time.

Putting time on your side

Start looking at your time and your schedule more carefully. Realize that time is an incredibly valuable commodity. What can you get rid of and are there ways to double up (but without becoming tangled up in excessive multi-tasking)?

Here are a few ideas:

- ✔ Dust the house or fold the laundry while you're talking on the phone.
- ✔ Cook extra meals on the weekend and put some in the freezer for later in the week.
- ✔ Create a basket with cleaning supplies you can carry around as you clean the house.

✔ Meet with someone over a walk. That way you get your exercise in at the same time.

✔ Book your appointments at the doctor, hairdresser, or other professional as the first one of the day. You won't spend as much time waiting.

✔ Always have something to do such as reading or planning at any appointment that's likely to involve a wait.

✔ Keep a list of things to do — whether on your computer or day planner — and review it everyday. Take on a small item whenever you have a few spare minutes. Just remember to review it often.

Recharging your batteries

You can take this efficiency stuff too far. You can't multitask every minute of the day. You also have to rejuvenate and recharge. Therefore, schedule some down time. You need breaks during the day. See Chapter 18 for information on meditation, which can help you benefit even more from down time.

You also need to take vacations. If you feel like you don't want to travel, that's fine, but you still need to get away sometimes. You can get away by scheduling a week without obligations. Be sure your week includes things like going to the movies, working in your garden, taking long walks, eating at your favorite restaurants, and other ideas that you enjoy. For more suggestions, see Chapter 16.

Kids and stress

Research on happiness indicates that parents are the least happy from the time their children are around 2 years of age until they reach adolescence. Why? Probably because raising children takes huge amounts of time and is incredibly stressful. That's not to say that people would be happier if they sent their kids to boarding school or never had them in the first place. Children bring much joy and meaning into one's life. But if you have kids, you can reduce the amount of stress they cause by setting limits on their activities and schedules, especially during the dark days of winter. Too many parents believe that their children are never happy or fulfilled unless they're engaged in a crushing number of activities — soccer, piano lessons, scouting,

marshal arts, baseball, football, swimming, and so on. Kids actually do better with a limited range of activities, and you as a parent can feel less stress at the same time. Yes, it's important to go to their games, but you don't need to attend every single practice. Spread the work around a little by forming a carpool group with other parents.

Children need to know how to amuse themselves without every minute scheduled and taken care of for them. By the way, they won't master this skill if you allow them to sit mindlessly in front of the TV or with video games hours on end. You can also reduce your stress by having your kids take on a reasonable number of household chores. Trust us; it's good for them!

Finding the lighter side

Humor is a great stress buster. When you feel overwhelmed, overworked, and overburdened, find a way to laugh at yourself or life in general. Stop taking everything so seriously. You won't get a gold medal for having the cleanest house, an always-balanced checkbook, or the best organized garage.

SAD doesn't seem especially funny, but you can inject humor into your life:

- Watch comedies.
- Read funny books.
- Go watch the monkeys at your local zoo for a while.
- Watch a group of 5-year-olds play T-ball.

Now, let's see; we need to say something funny here. After all, we can't conclude a section on humor without something funny. Did you hear the one about how many psychologists it takes to change a light bulb? Only one, but the bulb has to *want* to change . . . (sorry) . . .

Part IV
Changing SAD Behaviors

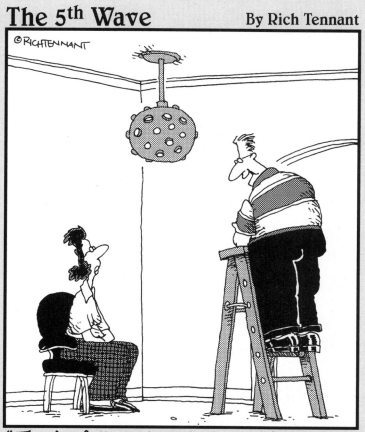

The 5th Wave   By Rich Tennant

"They're full spectrum bulbs, so it'll manage your seasonal affective disorder _and_ you'll learn how to dance."

In this part . . .

We cover the behavioral approaches to seasonal affective disorder (SAD). By changing some of your behaviors, you can change the way you feel.

First, we help you see if sleep problems are contributing to your SAD. Then we tell you about methods for improving sleep. Next you get info to help you get going again when SAD bogs you down. One of the ways to get going is through exercise, and you deal with un-motivating thoughts that can get in your way of exercising. Finally, we tell you how to start bringing fun back into your life.

Chapter 13

Sleep and SAD

Sleep refreshes and rejuvenates. Sleep helps repair the body and is critical to learning and memory. People with depression or seasonal affective disorder (SAD) often complain about problems with sleep. Folks with non-seasonally related depression often report not sleeping enough, but SAD sufferers typically say the opposite — that they sleep too much. Neither type of problem is much fun.

Sleep problems — either too little or too much — chronic fatigue, and day-time sleepiness can also be symptoms of a serious medical problem. Be sure to talk to your healthcare provider if you have consistent difficulty with sleeping or feel chronically tired. Common physical problems include

✔ **Alcohol, medications, and drugs:** All sorts of medications as well as illegal drugs and alcohol can all seriously disrupt sleep. Antidepressant medication sometimes improves sleep, but they can also disrupt sleep for some people. Discuss this option with your doctor.

✔ **Circadian rhythm disorders:** Essentially this disorder involves problems with the time of day or night you tend to fall asleep and awaken. Somehow your body and mind are out of synch with the sun and the moon and the stars. See Chapter 3 for more information on this problem.

✔ **Hormonal problems:** Women often have trouble staying asleep during early stages of menopause. Talk to your doctor if you have this problem.

✔ **Prostate problems:** An enlarged prostate can cause men to awaken multiple times per night to urinate. If you wake up more than once a night for this reason, consult your healthcare provider.

✔ **Restless leg syndrome:** People with restless leg syndrome have an uncontrollable urge to move their legs and feet. This syndrome can be quite distressing and interfere with sleep. Medication is available — talk to your doctor.

✔ **Sleep apnea:** This problem involves a short cessation of breathing followed by a rapid gulp of air. Many people are unaware they have this condition, so their partners are often the first ones to detect it. Most folks with sleep apnea also snore, but not all snorers have it. Sleep apnea is a serious problem because it can cause decreased oxygen to the brain and stress the heart — so if you suspect it, have it checked out.

In this chapter, we fill you in on how much sleep a person normally requires for optimal functioning. Sleep problems increase depressive symptoms, whether you're sleeping too much or too little. We also help you solve sleep disruptions of both types.

Determining the Sleep You Need

People require different amounts of sleep. Young babies may need almost 16 hours of sleep, toddlers about 12. Sleep experts believe that healthy adults do best on between seven to nine hours of sleep each night. If you get the right amount of sleep, you wake up feeling refreshed and active during the day.

So, how do you determine how much sleep is just enough for you? We have some steps for you to follow, but there are a couple of things to take into consideration first:

✔ **Are you experiencing SAD now?** The steps below to determine your sleep needs won't work for you if you're in the throes of a serious depressive episode (whether seasonal or non-seasonal). Wait until you feel better to try it.

✔ **Do you smoke or drink?** Don't drink coffee, cola drinks, alcohol, or smoke cigarettes for the week of this test. Also, don't take sleep-inducing medications during this test week. Cigarettes are stimulating, and alcohol can disrupt your sleep, so really try to give these things up for this week.

If you're a regular smoker, drinker, or take medication for sleeping, stopping for this exercise allows you to see how much sleep your body requires.

Why sleep?

Sleep is a complex process with many functions. Scientists study sleep by hooking electrodes to the skulls of people and recording brain wave activities. Several stages of brain activities correspond with stages of sleep:

↙ During the waking state, the brain has fast activity called the beta rhythm.

↙ When drowsy or relaxed, the brain slows to an alpha rhythm.

↙ In deep sleep the brain produces an even slower delta rhythm. During deep sleep, there's also a time in which the brain is active. This period is called REM (rapid eye movement) sleep and involves the sleeper being relatively still, with eyes moving rapidly behind closed lids and twitches of the mouth, fingers, and toes. This is the time of dreaming.

Sleeping is an adaptive response to conserve energy when food isn't available. Humans sleep after eating when dinner is over. Different animals sleep at different times depending on when food gathering takes place. Sleep also appears to be restorative and helps the immune system. You need sleep in order to perform complex tasks. Sleep seems to play some part in organizing and storing events into memory, and during sleep your blood pressure drops, breathing becomes slower, muscles are relaxed, and tissue growth and repair occur.

To find out how much sleep you need, for one full week, take the following steps:

1. **Decide what time you need to get up in the morning.**

   The time depends on your own schedule. Just make it the same time every day.

2. **Set your alarm clock for the time decided on in Step 1.**

   Get up when the alarm goes off! No snoozing or rolling over for ten more minutes!

3. **Don't take naps during the day.**

   No matter how tired you feel, resist the urge to nap. Most people find that napping is disruptive to their night sleep.

4. **Go to sleep at night when you feel tired — not before.**

   If you don't fall asleep within 15 minutes, get out of bed and do something else like read, watch TV, or surf the Internet.

5. **Return to bed when you're sleepy.**

Give this process some time. Your body tells you when you need to go to sleep. If you need more, go to bed earlier; if you need less you start to feel tired later.

6. **At the end of the week, tally up how much sleep you were getting the last two or three nights.**

That's likely to be how much you need. You'll know it's enough if you're feeling refreshed in the morning and have reasonable energy during the day. If you aren't feeling refreshed or drag through the day, you may need a little more sleep. After you've assessed how much sleep you need, be sure to adjust your schedule to set aside just that many hours every night. If you're getting nine hours or more of sleep and it doesn't feel like enough, check with your doctor.

Getting Up and Out of Bed

If you have SAD, sleep probably comes easily, too often, and lasts too long. Getting up is hard to do. Everyone has difficulty getting out of bed from time to time. We both like to hit the snooze button on winter mornings when it's dark and cold and squeeze in just a few more minutes of sweet sleep. Doing this means that we have to speed up our morning routine, or write one less page in our book that day. These aren't huge consequences.

But for some people, that snooze button and the oversleeping that results lead to missing appointments or being chronically late for work. Feeling behind schedule all the time increases stress and can make depression worse. (And having your boss upset with you doesn't help, either.) So, if you have SAD and you can't seem to get out of bed, jump-start your day with these strategies:

✔ **Get the alarm clock(s) that you need.** Some people need a very loud alarm clock, others do fine with clock radios. If you tend to turn the clock off and go back to sleep, here are a few suggestions:

- Put the alarm across the room.

- Get more than one alarm clock and put them in different spots in your room.

- Put a wind up alarm clock under a large cooking pan that's turned upside down.

- Get an alarm clock that actually falls off the table when it rings and rolls around the floor (yes, they really do make those).

The main idea here is to wake up and *get out* of bed — no matter what it takes to accomplish the goal.

✔ **Get enough sleep.** Most adults need about eight hours or so. But, if you don't get enough sleep on a night or two, get up anyway and make sure you have enough the next night. See "Determining the Sleep You Need" earlier in this chapter to determine if you get the sleep you need.

✔ **Watch out for caffeine, sleep aid drugs, nicotine, and alcohol.** These items all alter or interfere with sound sleep. Talk to your healthcare provider if you have concerns.

✔ **Simplify your morning routine.** In order to decrease stress, have your clothes out the night before. Pack your lunch and briefcase. Organize what you need and put everything in the same place before you go to bed.

✔ **Go to bed and get up at the same time every day.** The body does best with regular rhythms (see Chapter 3).

✔ **Try a dawn simulator.** This light turns on gradually before you wake up. You can also get a dawn simulator that provides bright light therapy for use after you awaken (see Chapter 5 for more info).

✔ **Let the sunshine in.** Open up the curtains, even a cloudy day provides some sunlight. During winter, especially at high latitudes, consider spending some time early in the morning using bright lights (see Chapter 5). And make sure your room and bathroom are well lit.

✔ **Get moving.** Turn up the music, stretch, walk in place, get your blood pumping. And try to get some exercise during the daytime, preferably outdoors (see Chapter 15).

✔ **Fuel up with oxygen.** Start with this little exercise:

   1. **Start with your arms at your side.**

   2. **Slowly raise your arms above your head while breathing in very deeply through your nose.**

   3. **Then slowly lower your arms down to your sides as you breathe out fully through your mouth.**

      Make the breath out firm and forceful.

   4. **Repeat four to five times.**

✔ **Take a shower, switch the water from hot to as cold as you can stand.** After your shower, rub yourself vigorously with a towel to get the blood pumping. Or splash your face with cold water.

✔ **Have a drink of cold water, a cup of coffee, or tea as soon as you wake up.** Caffeine in small amounts has been found to be harmless. Talk to your doctor if you have concerns or if you have high blood pressure.

✔ **Make a rule that after you're out of bed, you stay up.** You may want to go back to bed for just a few minutes, but that only makes it harder the next day. Keep moving and keep going, your fatigue is likely to pass.

When you're in an episode of SAD, you're likely to *feel* like you actually need more sleep. However, after you go beyond seven to nine hours, you actually compound your problems by sleeping more. Work hard to limit your sleep to a normal range and you're actually likely to find yourself feeling more rested within a week or two.

Falling Asleep and Staying Asleep

SAD can also be accompanied by problems falling asleep and waking in the middle of the night and not being able to fall back asleep. Often sleep finally comes shortly before the alarm goes off and makes getting out of bed even more difficult.

If you're having chronic trouble falling asleep or staying asleep, talk to your doctor and maybe your therapist Sleep medication is one approach, but generally isn't the best long-term solution. Ultimately acquiring good sleep habits usually helps the most.

> **Brenda** grew up in Louisiana and was diagnosed with SAD after moving to Philadelphia five years ago. She always had trouble falling asleep, but now with SAD, she finds herself tossing and turning night after night. She asks her doctor for some sleep medication. She finds herself depending on the medication to go to sleep, but she's still waking up around 3 a.m. Then she worries about going back to sleep. When the alarm finally goes off at 6:30 a.m, she's exhausted before her day starts.
>
> Brenda's doctor, concerned about her sleep, refers her to a sleep clinic. The sleep clinic rules out any physical problems and provides her with education on how she can improve her sleep. Brenda discovers that she's regularly spending too much time just before bed rushing around the house, cleaning, catching up on bills, and helping the kids with homework. Her stress and anxiety just before bed make it hard for her to sleep. She works to decrease the stress before bedtime by sticking to a schedule of chores and homework earlier in the evening.
>
> Brenda knew she needed some help with her sleep issues. Even after getting the sleep medication, when she continued to have problems, she went back to her doctor to address the issues. Don't assume that if your doctor gives you a prescription and it doesn't work that there's nothing else you can do. Brenda found that working on her pre-bedtime routine did the trick.

If your sleep problems aren't chronic (meaning they haven't been ongoing for weeks), you may need just a little extra help to get your ZZZs. If you want to try to get back into a routine of restful sleep, try the following suggestions:

- ✔ **Establish a bedtime routine.** If you have sleep problems, keeping to one routine is *imperative*. Gone are the days when you could stay up all night and sleep all day. Most adults can't easily switch sleeping shifts.

- ✔ **Switch off the stress.** Find a relaxing book or play soft music in the hour before bed. You don't want to be paying bills, writing a report, or yelling at the kids an hour before bed.

- ✔ **Consider taking a warm bath.** Turn off the phone; buy some bubbles or oils; relax for a while. Play soft music and light some scented candles.

- ✔ **Eat and drink.** While milk and cookies are okay, don't choose a big meal, caffeinated drinks, or alcohol.

- ✔ **Exercise.** If you can get out for an evening walk, that's great, but you don't want to wake your body up too much or you won't be able to fall asleep, so don't exercise right before going to bed.

- ✔ **Have an inviting place to sleep.** Invest in a good mattress, make sure that your room is dark, and purchase soft sheets. Buy new pillows if yours are less than great.

- ✔ **Dress for the job.** Wear comfortable clothing. Soft cotton or flannel pajamas are good choices.

- ✔ **Keep the room cool.** People generally sleep better when the room is cool. If you're cold, add blankets.

- ✔ **Keep the room quiet.** Although some people can go to sleep with soft music or television, changes in noise level can disrupt your sleep. You can buy sound machines that have soothing noises (white noises, ocean waves, wind, and babbling brooks) that help some people sleep better. Comfortable ear plugs may help, especially if you have thin walls, live in New York City, or have a noisy bed partner.

- ✔ **Practice relaxation or deep breathing techniques.** Get comfortable in your bed, lie on your back, place a hand on your tummy, and breathe in and out slowly. Imagine relaxing all the muscles and slowly sinking into your mattress (see Chapter 11 for more tips on relaxation).

After implementing all or most of the above steps and you're still struggling with sleep issues after several days, you definitely need to see your doctor. There's no need to suffer endlessly with sleeplessness!

Medications for sleep

Many over-the-counter medications and prescription medications exist for sleep problems. Whether prescription or not, sleeping pills aren't considered cures for insomnia. They all have side effects, and some of them can be addictive. Most sleep aids you find in the drug store aisles contain antihistamines, which are relatively safe but can cause drowsiness the next day. They may also interfere with the quality of your sleep.

Your medical provider may prescribe a short-acting sedative hypnotic, such as Ambien (zolpidem), Sonata (zaleplon), or Lunesta (eszopiclone). Rozerem (ramelteon) works on the melatonin (a hormone that affects sleep) receptors in the brain, but it isn't a narcotic. These drugs appear to be safer than older medications commonly used for sleep such as benxodiazepams, which could lead to dependence and impairment in memory. Nevertheless, even the newer medications have some risk of dependency. Side effects of these have included memory impairment and day-time drowsiness. Medications weren't designed for long-term use.

If you do take medications for sleep, follow the directions of your healthcare provider. You should also use the strategies in this book. For more information about sleep and insomnia, go to the Web site for the National Sleep Foundation: www.sleepfoundation.org.

Warning: A frightening, rare side effect of some sleep medications is what's known as *sleep driving.* Sleep driving is a more complicated and dangerous form of sleep walking in which people report no memory of getting up and going for a ride. A more common side effect of sleep medications involves waking up in the middle of the night and binge eating with no memory of having done so the following morning. Both reactions can be a little scary. Be sure to strictly follow your doctor's instructions when using sleep medications.

Thinking about Sleeping instead of Sleeping

When you have trouble going to sleep at night do you have nagging self-talk that starts to chatter in your head? Do you start thinking, "Oh this is terrible; I'll be beat tomorrow; I'm going to feel horrible all day." Or do you think, "I'll never fall asleep; I can't stand this." What does your self-talk say?

When those words and thoughts start chattering in the night, they can stir up unpleasant emotions. And these emotions can set off a series of physical responses that include an increased heart rate and a surge of adrenalin, a stimulating hormone. And you guessed it, these physical responses make it ten times more difficult to sleep. Therefore, the more upset you get about your sleeping problems, the more you can't sleep.

The opposite can also occur. Some people who stay in bed longer than they want start beating themselves up for not having any energy. Their self-talk might say, "I feel terrible, I can't be normal, I sleep too much and still feel lousy. I'm a lazy, no good person." Not exactly thoughts for putting you in a good mood to start the day.

In various chapters in this book (see especially Chapters 9 and 10), we provide information about how thoughts affect moods. Thoughts also affect sleep, sometimes rather profoundly. And you can use the same techniques described in those chapters to address your sleep disturbing thoughts.

One effective method to shutting down the self-talk is to acknowledge it and then change it. Writing those thoughts out or talking them over with a friend or therapist can help you see how your thoughts have been ruining your sleep and how to change them for the better.

Take a look at Savannah's story:

> **Savannah** is a 49-year-old bookkeeper who was divorced six years ago. She knows that the winter months have always been her least productive time of the year. Though never falling into a full-blown episode of SAD, Savannah consistently experiences the winter blues (see Chapter 2).
>
> This winter has been especially bitter cold, and Savannah finds herself struggling more than usual. Her new relationship has been going great, but her boyfriend now tells her that she's been increasingly irritable, lethargic, and, frankly, not a whole lot of fun to be around. He tells her that counseling may help, and she agrees.
>
> Savannah actually has a combination sleep problem — she often wakes up for hours, and on some nights she only sleeps for three or four hours. On other nights she sleeps for ten hours and feels like if she could just get an hour or two more sleep that she'd be okay. However, her counselor tells her that more sleep won't do the trick on such nights, and the nights with too little sleep aren't great either.
>
> So the counselor instructs Savannah to start noticing her thoughts that relate to sleep — those that occur while she's trying to go to sleep, those that start running through her head when she wakes up at 2:00 a.m., and those that tell her to sleep longer even though she's been sleeping for more than nine hours. She realizes that some of her thoughts sabotage her efforts to get a regular, balanced night's sleep while other thoughts can help counteract the self-sabotaging ones.

Savannah develops a simple chart that she keeps by her bed. In the chart she writes out the thoughts that are keeping her awake in one column, and then writes out thoughts that are more accurate and less sleep disrupting (called sleep-inducing thoughts). This process helps expose the irrationality of the thoughts and provides a less emotionally arousing alternative.

Take a look at Savannah's Sleep-Sabotaging and Sleep-Inducing Thoughts Form in Table 13-1 to see how she shut down her sleep robbing thoughts.

Table 13-1	Savannah's Sleep-Sabotaging Thoughts and Sleep-Inducing Thoughts Form
Sleep-Sabotaging Thoughts	*Sleep-Inducing Thoughts*
I really can't stand it when I don't sleep well.	That's catastrophizing. I "don't like" not sleeping well, but it's hardly the end of the world.
Just another hour of sleep, and I'll be okay; I don't want to get up!	True, I don't want to get up. But whenever I sleep more, I still feel crummy. I'm going to throw myself out of bed now.
It's 3:00 a.m., and I've been awake for an hour. I'll never go back to sleep. And if I don't, my day will be awful.	I don't know if I'll go back to sleep or not. If I don't go back to sleep, I have to remember what my counselor told me — I've survived many days on just a little sleep. It's uncomfortable, not *awful*.
If I don't get enough sleep, it feels like it could kill me.	Hmm, sort of unlikely. Again, a lack of sleep is uncomfortable, but it's totally survivable.
I just have to get to sleep; I've been tossing and turning for an hour and a half.	Actually, my counselor said to get up for a while if I don't fall asleep within 20 or 30 minutes. This break won't kill me and will teach my body to start falling asleep more consistently if I do go ahead and get up.

Now it's your turn. Follow these steps:

1. **Take a piece of paper and draw a table like Savannah's Sleep-Sabotaging and Sleep-Inducing Thoughts.**

2. **Jot down your sleep-sabotaging thoughts as soon as you notice them in your head.**

   You can write down the more reasonable thoughts (sleep-inducing thoughts) later if you want to. You're likely to find that over time, your sabotaging thoughts slowly reduce.

Sleep is important and very helpful. However, a few restless nights aren't horrible and you can get through a day or two without enough sleep. The paradox is that the more it is okay not to sleep, the more likely you will.

Chapters 9 and 10 give you a lot of ideas for tackling all types of negative thinking. If this exercise proves difficult for you, read those chapters first. Then go back and work on your sleep-disrupting thoughts.

Chapter 14

Fighting SAD by Getting Moving

. . . .

In This Chapter
▶ Thinking about doing

▶ Digging doing

▶ Solving immobilization with specific strategies

. . . .

Seasonal affective disorder (SAD) can immobilize you. Simple tasks and projects seem more complex and difficult, if not downright impossible. SAD symptoms include fatigue, a desire to sleep more, and decreased motivation. Unfortunately, when these symptoms keep you from doing your usual activities, depression deepens. The less you do, the less you feel like doing, and the guiltier you feel for not staying on top of your responsibilities.

Fortunately, this chapter provides an antidote. Get moving again. As your activity increases, you're very likely to notice your mood improving and your energy returning — studies prove it!

Mobilizing for Action

Negative thinking keeps you from taking actions that can help dig you out of your depression. So if you "think" you just can't do anything but pull the covers over your head, we ask you to think again.

It seems counterintuitive, but getting up, out, and moving are actually the best things you can do. To help get you where you need to go, you need to assess where you have do-nothing thinking. Do-nothing thinking tells you that you can't take action, that you are overwhelmed, and that you should just stay put and do nothing. In this section, we show you how to defeat such defeatist thinking. Then you'll be prepared to get moving again, and your moods will lighten up as a result.

Reginald, a book editor, illustrates how this process of defeating do-nothing thinking works.

Reginald moved to upstate New York and started his new career as an editor last summer. He enjoys the fast pace of the publishing business and excitement of learning new material. Reginald makes friends quickly and is delighted by an early fall snowstorm. The city shuts down, and he enjoys his first "snow day" by hanging out and watching the news between bouts of snow shoveling. He calls his friends back in Atlanta, where he grew up, and brags about the drifts of up to five feet.

After a few weeks of snow, ever shortening days, ice storms, and cold, Reginald's enthusiasm begins to drift downward. He feels like he's running out of gas and decides to take vitamins. That doesn't seem to help, and he starts spending many weekends sleeping in, watching television, and avoiding his new friends. His townhouse is getting to be a mess — dishes pile in the kitchen, and unopened mail gathers dust on the desk.

An old friend visits from Atlanta and is shocked by the change in Reginald. Reginald explains that he feels horrible. He can't get out of bed; he's showing up late at work, and he derives no pleasure from his job. For the first time in his life, Reginald's checkbook isn't balanced, and he receives late charges on his credit cards. He ignores his work responsibilities and seems totally stalled. He thinks, "Every thing feels overwhelming to me. I can't handle this, maybe I should quit and move back home."

Reginald goes to his doctor who gives him a complete physical that reveals no physical, obvious causes for his low moods. His doctor then suggests that he may be suffering from SAD. He refers Reginald to a psychologist who specializes in the treatment of this disorder. Reginald tells the psychologist about his fatigue, lack of energy, and overall boredom. The psychologist reviews Reginald's symptoms and agrees that he may have a case of SAD, although technically it would take another season of suffering to know for sure (see Chapter 2 for more information about the diagnosis of SAD). Here is their discussion:

Psychologist: So, Reginald, one of the best things you can do for SAD is to increase your activities.

Reginald: Yeah, I know that's a good idea, but I really don't feel up to it.

Psychologist: Okay, let's put that on the back burner. Tell me a little about what's making you feel down.

Reginald: I feel horrible about work. I'm not getting anything done at work or at home. I've let my checkbook go; I haven't cleaned my apartment in four weeks; I could go on and on.

Psychologist: That's quite a list. What thoughts go through your mind when you think about doing one of those things on your list?

Reginald: Well, I think that I don't have any energy. I can't get started. If I do start, I'll just fail. I'm beginning to think I'm just a lazy person. I don't feel like doing anything. And then I think if I rest up, I'll get the energy to do something eventually.

Psychologist: Has resting more done that for you?

Reginald: Actually, no. I've been getting more tired everyday.

Psychologist: That's a very common thought that stops people in their tracks. You *think* you'll feel better with more rest, but you find that your fatigue merely deepens.

Reginald: You're right. No matter how much sleep I get, I feel incredibly tired and drained. But what can I do about it?

Psychologist: That's a very good question; I'm glad you asked it. I'm sure you feel overwhelmed.

Reginald: You got that right. My to-do list is so long that it almost makes me want to cry.

Psychologist: That makes sense. Anyone can feel snowed under by a huge, long to do list. So I'm going to recommend that we only tackle a couple of items at first and build momentum from there.

Reginald: That's fine, but I just don't think I'm up to the task.

Psychologist: Hang in there with me for a little bit. For starters, I recommend challenging your "do-nothing" thinking. Let's have you start by filling out the Defeating Do-Nothing Thinking Form.

The form is actually very simple to complete. Reginald's psychologist noted a few items as they chatted and helped Reginald get his chart started.

Here are the steps for the form, and a portion of Reginald's completed form is shown in Table 14-1:

1. **List your do-nothing thoughts in the left-hand column.**

2. **In the right column, write down thoughts to counteract your do-nothing thoughts.**

In developing your counteracting thoughts, consider these questions:

- What would I tell a friend who had thoughts like these?

- Have I ever been able to overcome this sort of thought before?

- Is my do-nothing thought illogical or distorted in any way?

- Is my do-nothing thought just based on feelings instead of sound evidence?

- Am I simply labeling myself in an unhelpful way?

- Is it possible I can just put my do-nothing thought to the test?

Table 14-1	Reginald's Defeating Do-Nothing Thinking Form
Do-Nothing Thoughts	*Counteracting Thoughts*
I don't have enough energy to do anything.	Actually, my energy will just drain away if I don't do anything. Truth is, I think it's possible I'll have more energy if I start doing things.
I need to rest up before I get started.	That thought has just made things worse.
I don't feel like doing anything.	Since when do you have to feel like doing something in order to do it? Maybe I'll start feeling like doing things if I do things first!
I'm a lazy person.	That's an unhelpful label. I have only been like this since my SAD took hold. Just because I have SAD doesn't mean I'm lazy.
If I try, I'll just fail.	And if I don't try, it's automatic failure. I can test this thought out by trying and seeing what happens.

Reginald finds the form useful. By filling it out, he realizes that his thoughts are useless mind chatter that stop him before he gets started. He decides to follow his psychologist's advice and start keeping an activity log (see the next section "Taking Action").

You don't necessarily need a therapist to defeat your do-nothing thinking. Take a notebook and draw a table like Table 14-1. Fill in any self-defeating, do-nothing thoughts that you hear rambling through your mind. Then go through our list of suggested questions for helping you come up with counteracting thoughts. See Chapters 9 and 10 for more information about how to deal with negative thinking.

Taking Action

This section is where the rubber meets the road. It's time to move from negative thinking to positive actions. The more you do, the more you feel like doing. When you don't get things done, you're likely to scold yourself. When you put yourself down that way, you squash any motivation you may have had. A negative cycle ensues in which inaction leads to dark moods that lead to even more inaction.

On the other hand, when you go ahead and take action, a "positive spiral" gets started. Like the expression, "one good deed deserves another," it's also true that "one small action leads to another." Which brings us to our first principle — start small. In the following sections, you discover the steps to getting going. The process of restarting your life includes taking small steps, making sure your activities give you a balance of pleasure and mastery, and keeping track of what you do.

Taking baby steps

An old, but very funny movie portrayed a psychiatrist who wrote a best selling book called *Baby Steps*. Although the psychiatrist's advice seemed absurdly simplistic, the principle is actually quite sound. When tackling SAD, you should take things one small step at a time. That's because if you look at everything that you may wish to do in the future all at once, your tasks will easily overwhelm you — sort of like imagining that you must eat all the food you plan to eat in the next year at one sitting or thinking that you must walk all the steps you're going to walk in your lifetime, this week. Such images can stop a charging rhino in its tracks (that is, if rhinos could contemplate the future).

Therefore, whenever your mind tells you that a task is too overwhelming, the key is to break it down into small, baby steps. Then start doing each step, one at a time. Revisit Reginald and see how his therapist helps him get started on the little things:

> Reginald returns to his therapist the following week. He tells him that his mood is a bit better and he has been getting to work on time. He still has a long list of undone things. Here's their conversation:
>
> **Psychologist:** I'm delighted that you found working with the Defeating Do-Nothing Thinking Form useful and that your mood has improved a bit. What have you noticed in the past week that seems most helpful?
>
> **Reginald:** I found myself challenging my thinking. I have some hope that I'll get back on track, and I did get better about getting up on time.
>
> **Psychologist:** Great. At the beginning of each session, I like to set an agenda. It's easy to get off track, and the agenda helps both of us to stay focused on an issue. Of course, if something comes up and we need to switch, the agenda isn't written in stone. So, what would you like to talk about and work on today?
>
> **Reginald:** You know, I'm still pretty stuck with a lot of things undone at home. My house is a mess, and I told you my bills are stacked up. I get my paycheck deposited into my checking account, but I haven't balanced it since last July. Then of course those deadlines are getting closer for my job. It's just too much.

Psychologist: I hear you say that you have too much to do. When you think about everything at once, you become overwhelmed. How about we pick one area to concentrate on and set the others aside for now?

Reginald: You know, it's hard for me to even pick one thing. By the way, I also notice that I am having trouble making even the easiest decisions.

Psychologist: That's pretty common in people with SAD. The brain feels sort of mushy. Am I right?

Reginald: Absolutely. But, you know, I'm thinking that I really need to get my bills and checkbook under control. That's costing me money, and I feel horrible when I have to pay late fees because I'm so lazy that I can't even make the effort to write a lousy check.

Psychologist: Sounds like the checkbook would be a useful place to start.

Reginald: Yeah, but it still feels overwhelming.

Psychologist: Let's break that task down into baby steps. Let's make a list of all the steps that are involved with balancing your checkbook and paying your bills.

Reginald: Well, first there's checking off all the checks that have cleared and those that haven't. Second, I suppose is checking off all the deposits and making sure they're in my check registry. That information is all online I guess. I'm starting to feel a little overwhelmed.

Psychologist: Okay, let's stop here. Do you think it would be possible to spend 15 minutes each day on the task of recording cleared checks until that part is finished. And then 15 minutes each day until all of the deposits are recorded?

Reginald: Well, I suppose so, but what about getting it all to reconcile and paying all my bills?

Psychologist: Are any of your bills overdue? If so, how many?

Reginald: Well, just one actually.

Psychologist: Could you pay that one and then start on the first task? You can deal with reconciling the checkbook and the rest of the bills a little later.

Reginald: I guess that makes sense. I can do that.

If you, like Reginald, have felt immobilized by the size of the chores that lie ahead, you're likely to make better headway if you break the task down into small, doable steps. *Consistency of effort* is the key to reaching your goals. Stop thinking about the entire undertaking all at once.

To give you a concrete idea of what we are talking about, we've listed a couple of large, easily overwhelming tasks below. Then we break them down into more manageable steps.

Cleaning the house

If you think you're the first person with SAD to have a disheveled house, you're wrong. It's hard to clean your house when getting out of bed seems difficult. But you can break the task down.

Consider these options:

- ✔ Decide to do only one room each day. There are no rules or laws that say you must clean the entire house in a single day.
- ✔ Gather all your cleaning materials in a bucket or container so you aren't running back and forth to get supplies.
- ✔ Do just one task each day. You can dust, vacuum, clean a toilet, get rid of some clutter, or put a few things away.
- ✔ Decide to clean for just 20 minutes per day.
- ✔ Clean during television commercials.

Writing a paper, work report, or a book

People love to put off writing. As professional book writers, we've had to work hard to overcome procrastination on this task. Over the years, we've learned a few tricks.

Breaking the work into baby steps can be done in various ways, depending on the nature of the project:

- ✔ List any and all ideas that you may want to incorporate. Don't censor your ideas, just jot them down.
- ✔ Pick the ideas you definitely want to keep, toss the others.
- ✔ Outline the project. You may wish to outline one portion at a time.
- ✔ A page a day keeps the editors at bay. Make a rule to write one page per day. If you feel like writing more, great! You can even decide a paragraph each day will do. Remember to be consistent.

Succeeding and pleasing

When you engage in an activity, you may feel two types of emotions:

- ✔ **Mastery:** Tasks that feel like challenges typically evoke a sense of mastery because you feel you've accomplished something that took effort.
- ✔ **Pleasure:** Other tasks simply feel good — like eating Belgian chocolate — it doesn't take much effort, but it may induce pleasurable sensations.

Some tasks — like taking a great photograph — feel like success and pleasure at the same time. Reginald (discussed in the preceding sections) started his activities with a focus on mastery.

> **Reginald,** during his subsequent visit, is pleased to tell his psychologist that not only did he balance his checkbook, but also he paid his bills. Like Reginald, you may very well find that you accomplish more than you initially set out to do. Remember that completing small goals adds up. Check out the therapy discussion this time:
>
> **Reginald:** Now I am ready to tackle the rest of my procrastinated projects. I feel pretty great about balancing my checkbook. What next?
>
> **Psychologist:** Hold on, take a breath. It's wonderful that you mastered your checkbook. Now, let me ask you about another important part of getting better. What are you doing during the week for fun?
>
> **Reginald:** Are you kidding? I'm so far behind at work I can't even begin to start having fun.
>
> **Psychologist:** I'm writing you a prescription. The prescription is for you to put a little fun back into your life. I want you to schedule a few activities that involve pleasure, just like you scheduled a bit of time to balance your checkbook.

You should have a balance of both pleasurable and mastery activities. And you'll probably find that some tasks give you both a sense of accomplishment as well as pleasure. Don't neglect pleasurable activities. For more ideas about having fun and pleasurable activities, be sure to check out Chapter 16.

Tracking your actions

Keeping an activity log is one of the best first steps you can take if you have a severe case of SAD and you're neglecting important responsibilities or chores. The technique is straightforward and fairly simple.

An activity log simply involves listing your main activities day-by-day. You also indicate how each activity made you feel in order to help you know what activities do for your moods. This information helps you plan more activities that improve your moods and reduce those that don't. Reginald discusses this task with his psychologist and then keeps a log:

> **Reginald:** You want me to keep a log of my activities. What good will that do?
>
> **Psychologist:** It's funny; keeping track of what you do actually gets you to do more and increases positive feelings.
>
> **Reginald:** Really? I hate to sound skeptical, but . . .

Psychologist: No, it's good you question things, Reginald. I welcome that. There have been studies that compared various treatments for depression. And surprisingly, one of the most effective strategies is to simply get people moving again. Furthermore, these studies show that tracking your activities helps you stay on track.

Reginald: Well, I guess I have nothing to lose by trying it.

Psychologist: Here's the form. How about you try this for two weeks and then we can see how it has gone for you?

Reginald: Deal.

In Table 14-2, you see Reginald's log of how this process works. You can also find a blank form of Table 14-2 in Appendix A of this book.

Here are the steps for completing an activity log:

1. **Get out your notebook and write down each day in a column on the left side of a page (you can also use a day planner if you prefer).**

2. **Schedule one neglected activity for each day — make it a small activity at first!**

3. **After you complete the activity, write down how it went and how you feel about accomplishing it.**

Table 14-2	Reginald's Activity Log	
Day	*Activity*	*Outcome*
M	Stopped by the grocery store after work.	Mostly doing this activity gave me a sense of mastery. I finally did something useful.
T	Finally finished editing two books that were running behind.	This activity was amazingly pleasurable. There was some sense of accomplishment, but it was really so easy.
W	Spent 20 minutes cleaning my apartment.	I was surprised I could accomplish that much in that short amount of time. It inspires me to do more.
Th	I called my folks.	It was good catching up with them; I know how much connecting means to them.
F	I scheduled a dentist appointment.	That felt good; I've been putting that off forever.

(continued)

Day	Activity	Outcome
Sa	I went cross-country skiing with some guys from work.	That was pure fun.
Su	I cleaned my apartment for 30 minutes.	Hey, the place is shaping up a little. I think I'll do more tomorrow. It even felt a little pleasurable in addition to giving me a sense of accomplishment.

Table 14-2 *(continued)*

Reginald finds that simply keeping track of his activities improves his mood. He no longer thinks of himself as a lazy person. He and his psychologist continue their work, and Reginald gets better. He discovers more about SAD and knows that he'll prepare for the following winter. At the end of the ski season, he buys cross-country skis. And he's already started a savings account for a winter cruise to the Caribbean.

When you write about your outcome, think about how much sense of mastery and/or pleasure you experienced with the activity. You may even find it useful to rate mastery and pleasure on a 10-point scale.

If negative thinking starts to get in your way of carrying out an activity log, work through the section above, "Taking Action." In addition, you may find that you can get moving by merely noticing those negative thoughts and commanding your body to start moving anyway.

If you're unable to get yourself moving with an activity log, we strongly urge you to consider getting professional help.

Problem Solving with S.O.C.C.E.R.

SAD has another way of immobilizing you. When problems arise, dark moods easily cloud your mind and keep you from finding an effective solution to even simple problems. People with SAD report problems concentrating, overwhelming feelings of fatigue, and problems with procrastination. SAD can stall thoughts and make choices and decisions more difficult. Studies show that when people are down in the dumps, they have trouble solving life's little and big problems. So, how do you deal with this? Play soccer and score a solution!

Taking a vacation from SAD

Particularly useful actions against SAD are activities that increase your exposure to sunlight and the outdoors. Whether you walk, jog, ice skate, or ski, getting active outdoors can brighten your moods and increase your exposure to helpful light (see Chapter 5 for more info about the role of light in SAD). Also see Chapters 15 and 16 for more ideas about various types of winter activities.

Many people who suffer from SAD find that taking a vacation in the winter months improves their moods. Take your winter vacation somewhere other than Alaska or Seattle if you have SAD. The tropics make a better choice.

For a couple of weeks prior to leaving you can plan and anticipate the enjoyable activities. While on vacation, you benefit from getting away from work pressures, you get a lot of sunshine, and you see and learn about interesting people and places. Or perhaps you just sit on a beautiful warm beach and read trashy novels. Either way, your moods lift. And when you return, your fresh memories may just keep you warm until spring.

You can save a lot of money if you're willing to make your travel plans at the last minute. Cruise lines offer deeply discounted packages for passengers willing to hop on with little notice.

Being pampered in the sunshine almost certainly gives you a reprieve from SAD. However, such trips aren't a complete cure. If you have SAD, you need to also employ some of the other ideas recommended throughout this book when you return.

If problem solving becomes an issue for you, this technique can help clear away the clouds in your mind allowing you to reach a solution. We call this problem-solving strategy S.O.C.C.E.R:

1. **Get out a big sheet of paper or a white board to write down your thoughts and ideas.**

   Be creative. Don't censor. Let your thoughts and ideas flow.

2. **Define your problem.**

   $\underline{S}$ stands for *situation*. Include information about how the problem came about, how it makes you feel, how important the problem is to you, and any other relevant information. Be as detailed as possible. Describe the problem thoroughly.

3. **List all the possible solutions to your problem.**

   $\underline{O}$ means *options*. What are all of the possible solutions to your problem? Be creative and include all ideas, great or small. Discuss your problem with other people who you trust, gather information, explore *all* imaginable alternatives.

4. Consider all of the options and the most likely consequences for each.

<u>C</u> (the first C) is for *consequences*. Some consequences will be so unacceptable that you can immediately rule out the option. Of course you won't know for sure what may happen, but take your best guess.

5. Pick one of the options to carry out.

<u>C</u> (number two) refers to making a *choice*.

6. Make a plan to get yourself through your choice.

<u>E</u> is the *emotional* plan to enact your choice. The plan can include getting support from others, getting professional help, practicing relaxation strategies, or rehearsing what you're going to do with someone else.

7. Carry out the plan, and then look at the results.

<u>R</u> means *run, review,* and *revise*. Review or evaluate the effectiveness. If you need to, go back and change or revise your plan.

Now that you know the steps for S.O.C.C.E.R., you can use this problem-solving technique whenever you feel stuck or unable to come up with a solution to a life problem. You don't even have to be depressed!

It's not unusual to consider the possibility of relocating to a sunnier or lighter location if you have SAD. Places closer to the equator have more daylight in the winter months, and those locations often have better weather so you can spend more time outside. When the move makes sense, it can be a very reasonable option.

But, you may not be able to contemplate the enormity of a move. Moving involves tremendous effort, planning, and persistence, with or without SAD. That's pretty hard to accomplish when you can hardly get out of bed! But sometimes circumstances come together that make moving an option. At that time, S.O.C.C.E.R can help break the problem down and make reaching a decision more manageable. Consider Ashley's situation:

Ashley grew up in a suburb of Detroit. She married her high school sweetheart Craig, had two kids, and lived only a few miles from where she was born. Her husband was employed for 25 years at an automobile company, and she worked at a local hospital. They were financially comfortable.

But, Ashley hates winter. Hating winter is a big problem when you live in Michigan. Ashley has been treated for SAD on and off for about the last 10 years. She tried multiple antidepressant medications but didn't like the side effects. Therapy seems to work for a while, but when it gets dark at 4:30 p.m. and the thermometer doesn't break freezing for months, she feels horrible. She doesn't even consider relocation. Her family is in Michigan, and she wouldn't ever leave them. Never.

The automobile industry in Detroit has crumbled. Ashley's oldest son moves out of state. Craig's company offers a buyout if he agrees to quit his job. At the same time, the hospital where she works is considering some layoffs as well.

So, it's November — Ashley and her husband are faced with a decision. They can stay in Michigan and hope that the car business improves (which it may) or they can take the offer. If they do take the offer, they can either remain in Michigan or they can move somewhere with longer, brighter days. At first, Ashley feels frozen with fear at the idea of tackling such a huge decision. Her symptoms of SAD darken with the extra stress of this problem.

Ashley recalls learning about the S.O.C.C.E.R. problem-solving technique from her therapist. So she gets out a white board, and they begin the process:

1. **(S) Situation — Describe the problem thoroughly.**

   The economy here has been deteriorating. Craig has an offer that might be best to take. The good thing about his offer is that it would give us health insurance until we qualify for Medicare. My hospital actually could lay me off. But I love Michigan in spite of the harsh winters and the SAD that usually comes with it for me. My daughter lives here and so do a lot of my friends and family.

2. **(O) Options — Brainstorm the possibilities.**

   - Craig could take the buyout and look for a job here while I hope for the best at the hospital.

   - We could look for jobs in a sunnier state.

   - We could probably simplify our lives and live on our 401(k)s and other savings and small pensions — while remaining here or moving.

   - Craig could say no to the buyout and hope the company turns around; there are signs that it could.

   - We could put up our house for sale and decide what to do after we see what it sells for.

   - We could take a vacation and check some other states out. Our cousins live in Arizona — that's always seemed a little appealing to me.

3. **(C) Consequences — List the likely outcomes.**

   - Odds are if he looks for a job here, he isn't going to find something that feels like a good fit or has similar benefits in this area. And the situation at my hospital is looking pretty grim. Chances are that I will be in the layoff group or if I stay, my job will get a whole lot more stressful.

- Craig's skills are good enough to find something in another state. I can always find a job elsewhere with no problem. But I just don't feel ready yet. And I don't know enough about other places.

- We could cut back a lot financially if we really had to. But I know us; we like to spend money and travel a lot.

- The auto industry might turn around, but Craig's job is likely to have an oversupply of workers for some time to come. The turn-around is going to take a while.

- Putting our house up for sale keeps our options open. We could still do whatever we want. But it sure feels like a scary thing to do.

- I do like the idea of visiting Arizona. We can check out the housing market and the job market at the same time. But still, I get butter-flies in my stomach just thinking about moving.

4. (C) Choice — Select the best alternative(s).

First, we're going to take a much-needed vacation and visit our cousins in Arizona. We might also check out New Mexico on the same trip. We'll look at some new houses — we love doing that anyway. And we will look at the want ads in the paper. Then we're going to put our house up for sale. I am pretty sure we'll follow that with a decision to move, but these options keep all the doors open. The whole thing makes me pretty nervous though.

5. (E) Emotional Plan — Strategize how to pull it off from an emotional standpoint.

The trip part is easy. But selling the house is going to be a lot tougher. We have a lot of history here. And there is so much stuff! Over the past 25 years we've thought about moving, but we both love our home, and the thought of selling it to strangers is difficult.

But we've gone over the options thoroughly. Taking the vacation and selling the house are definitely the things to do. We can capture memories with photographs. We can break the task down into small steps each weekend. My friend recently opened up a thrift shop and would love to come over and help get rid of some of our stuff. We have a lot of friends who would be willing to help us, too. I think I'll kick this around with my therapist as well. He has said that moving to a sunnier location might really help my SAD. I need to ponder the positives in all of this — there really are quite a few.

6. **(R) Run, review, revise — carry out your plan, see how it went, and consider revision if need be.**

    Wow, the vacation went great! And we learned so much — especially about New Mexico! They have a dynamic new company there that makes small jet aircrafts and could offer my husband a job in a heartbeat. The house is on the market, but no bites yet. We may have to revise the game plan a little and consider dropping the price more than we'd like. But I can already tell that a move is going to be the best thing for us to do.

Ashley and Craig find the S.O.C.C.E.R. problem-solving strategy very helpful. Before writing everything out, they felt frozen in dealing with their complicated problem. But as they took the problem apart, step by step, they realized that they had more options than they'd thought and that the outcomes were likely to be okay.

Chapter 15

Exercising into a Good Mood

*I*f you've been awake and alive in the last ten years, you probably have heard the message — exercise more. But can exercise really help you with your seasonal affective disorder (SAD)? Research says yes. In this chapter, you discover the relationship between exercise, mood, and overall health. Most people agree that exercise is good for the body and mind. That's not where most folks get stuck.

The problem is finding the motivation and commitment to maintaining exercise as a regular part of your life. In this chapter, you can find the willpower and develop an exercise plan you can live with through a variety of options for exercise.

Adding Up the Benefits of Exercise

An increasing number of studies have shown that exercise improves your mood to cheer you up. Research also shows that exercise improves *serious* problems with mood as found in major depressive disorder and SAD.

But exercise does much more than improve mood, important as that may be. Exercise has been shown to ameliorate non-seasonal depression as well as SAD. Sadly, though, many folks don't exercise much at all, and those people who do exercise often allow it to drop off in the winter months. So, it's time to try and get you motivated. Check out exercise's well-known benefits:

✔ Studies indicate that exercise is likely to make you live longer (and healthier while you're doing it).

✔ You may reduce your risks of breast cancer.

✔ Your body heals faster after injury.

✔ Exercise raises your good cholesterol (known as HDL).

✔ Your sleep is likely to improve (see Chapter 13).

✔ You can reduce your chances of adult onset diabetes (Type-2).

✔ Exercise is related to fewer strokes.

✔ Your memory may improve with exercise, though more so for people in middle age and beyond.

✔ Your sexual function may improve, more so for folks aged 40 or older.

✔ Your immune system is stimulated.

✔ Your risk for various cancers may go down.

✔ Your balance improves, resulting in less risk of falling.

✔ Your bones remain stronger.

✔ Exercise saves you money — your overall medical costs are likely to decline.

Exercise is especially helpful for seniors for increased endurance, strengthened bones, and maintained independence.

A study conducted in Russia (where they have more than their fair share of SAD) found that exercise and light therapy worked about equally well in treating SAD. Not only that, both treatments resulted in weight loss — a common problem experienced by SAD sufferers. Furthermore, both treatments started working in only a week or so. Researchers in Finland also have suggested possible value in combining exercise and light therapy. Such a combination does seem like a good idea, and it's readily accomplished. You can either exercise indoors with bright lights (see Chapter 5) or you can exercise outdoors.

Minding Your Motivation

Working exercise into your life as a regular routine may sound daunting to you. That's probably even more the case if you're already in the throes of an episode of SAD. In fact, you may want to be in a good state of mind prior to undertaking exercise. However, even if you're currently experiencing SAD, you can start increasing your exercise. To some extent, believing that you should wait until you feel better to start exercising is putting the cart before the horse. Exercise can help you feel better even when you're feeling down!

Endorphins: One of the ways exercise helps

The brain generates a substance called endorphins that may be responsible for much of the benefits from exercise. Endorphins create a sense of well being, pleasure, and reduced feelings of pain and distress. They work a little like opiates such as heroin and morphine, but they're naturally produced, legal, and good for you. Additional benefits of endorphins include improved circulation, neutralized toxic substances, and reduced stress.

Scientists are still studying exactly how endorphins work and the various benefits they have for the body. By the way, you can also increase endorphins by eating chocolate, eating highly spiced foods, and having sex. Of course there are limits on how much you can turn to those sources to increase your levels of endorphins.

You can battle the lack of willpower or motivation in two main ways:

✔ **Forget about willpower:** The first battle is to realize that willpower doesn't exist in the first place. What? That's right; psychologists have never been able to come up with a measure of some internalized store of willpower. So don't wait around looking for willpower. You won't find willpower locked in your brain or stocked on the grocery shelves.

Instead, start challenging your thinking. You can feel *naturally* motivated (seemingly have more willpower) when you figure out how to confront and challenge your self-defeating thinking.

✔ **Take baby steps:** Gradually work your way into an exercise routine. And that approach is probably safer anyway because if you're starting in an out-of-shape condition, you don't want to push your body too fast and too far.

Before you start any exercise program, consult your doctor and get the all clear. Even limited exercise is unadvisable for a few people. For example, if you have asthma, you can have difficulty with aerobic exercise or cold air. Please check it out and be sure to stop if you have any trouble breathing or experience significant pain.

If you do have a physical condition that interferes with exercise, consider getting a referral to a physical therapist or an exercise physiologist. These medical professionals can work with your healthcare provider to come up with a safe exercise plan.

Breaking down resistance to exercise

The idea of exercise may not sound too appealing to you. The very idea may even feel overwhelming, especially if you're currently depressed. However, *not appealing* and *overwhelming* are concepts being thrown at you by a negative, possibly depressed mind. Such thoughts don't represent reality; they're only thoughts. And the way to overcome such thoughts is to take a hard look at them. Then spend a little time actively challenging or disputing those thoughts.

> **Brian** is an investment banker living in Toronto, Canada. He has had four prior episodes of SAD in the past six years and is feeling his usual winter blues even though it's only early October. His doctor has told him that he is pre-diabetic and really needs to start exercising. Brian decides to try bright light therapy, and he's feeling a bit better after about ten days. However, he still feels a little lethargic, and he knows exercise can help further improve his mood as well as help deal with his other health problems.

> But the moment Brian thinks about exercise, he feels defeated. He hears thoughts running through his head such as *I hate exercise; It's too cold to exercise; I'm feeling too low to succeed at exercising.*

> Brian happens to pick up a copy of *Seasonal Affective Disorder For Dummies* and decides to give the Defeating De-motivating Thinking Exercise a try. After he does, he succeeds in making important baby steps and slowly but surely increases his exercise. His blood sugar levels gradually decline, his good cholesterol improves, and his low moods start to disappear.

Brian's thoughts stood in his way of exercising. Table 15-1 lays out his thoughts that just happen to be among the most common thoughts reported when thinking about starting an exercise program. We call those thoughts *de-motivating thoughts*. Then Brian works at developing more reasonable ways of thinking that may help jumpstart his efforts. These thoughts are called — you guessed it — motivating thoughts.

Table 15-1	Defeating De-motivating Thoughts
De-motivating Thoughts	*Motivating Thoughts*
It's too cold to exercise.	Sure it's cold outside, but I can either start my exercise inside or just dress right for it.
I can't imagine exercising when I'm this depressed.	That's just my depressed mind talking. I'll start small and slowly build up from there.
It just isn't *me* to exercise.	That's only because it's the way I've looked at myself and exercise in the past. I can let it *become* me.

De-motivating Thoughts	Motivating Thoughts
I don't have enough time as it is; I can't possibly exercise.	Yes, it feels that way. But the fact is, I spend an hour or more watching television most evenings. I could spend half of that time exercising.
I don't like exercise.	I can't argue with that. But maybe I can try some activities that other people seem to like that I haven't tried before. Besides, I don't have to *love* it; all I have to do is find it tolerable. If I keep at it, everyone says it becomes fun.
I can't even get out of bed in the morning; how can I possibly exercise.	Now my mind is really trying to trick me. Fact is, I *do* get out of bed. It's hard, but I do it. And I can start with small steps. And just because I'm not really a morning person, doesn't mean I can't exercise later in the day.
Exercising in the cold can harm your health or your lungs.	I had to check this thought out with my doctor. He said that those ideas are myths. He told me to just dress warmly and get out there!

Brian's list of motivating and de-motivating thoughts merely represents some of the most common ways you can defeat yourself before you even get started. You need to listen to what *your* mind is specifically telling you. Write down any de-motivating thoughts you have on a sheet of paper divided into columns, just like in Table 15-1. Then see if you can come up with an alternative, more reasonable view that may help get you going.

If you struggle with the exercise in Table 15-1, read Chapters 9 and 10. Then go back and apply the knowledge from those chapters to this exercise.

Taking baby steps into exercise

You need to start your exercise program in small steps — don't try running three miles the first time out! Besides, you resist less if you start slowly. Then you very gradually increase the time and effort you put into your program.

You may have heard several different recommendations for exercise: A minimum of 20 to 30 minutes a day at least three days a week or an hour or so four or five times a week. However, studies have demonstrated that virtually any amount of exercise is better than none. And you can increase your time very slowly. You may be surprised by how much you end up doing (and liking), but again, anything is better than nothing.

Working out in your mind?

You've probably heard about placebos — the sugar pills often used in experiments to see if potent medications work the way they're supposed to work. You aren't told if you're receiving a real drug or a dummy pill (placebo) to see whether the real drug has an effect. Sometimes, you get about the same benefit from a placebo that you do with the real drug. This effect is called the placebo effect. It's based on the fact that when you believe in something, there's often a benefit.

Well, what do placebos have to do with exercise? Researchers at Harvard found a group of 84 hotel housekeepers. Housekeepers work fast and hard. Some of the housekeepers were told that the exercise they got while cleaning hotel rooms was enough to keep them fit. Others weren't told anything. After 4 weeks, the housekeepers who were told they were working out on the job lost about two pounds, lowered their blood pressure, and showed lower levels of body fat. This study provides evidence that positive *beliefs* about your exercise and fitness levels may in fact benefit your body. Ahhhh, the power of positive thinking!

 Small changes in your daily routine can add up to 20 or 30 minutes a day. For example, walk the stairs instead of taking the elevator, park a few spots down, walk around while you're on the phone, take a few laps around the mall, take a walk at lunch time, or balance on one foot while doing the dishes.

Exercising Away SAD

This book isn't a book on how to exercise. You can find a lot of help for that at your local bookstore, and we're also pretty sure there are a ton of *For Dummies* books on various forms of exercise. But, you can do a few types of exercise and take a few tips about exercise that are particularly relevant to SAD sufferers.

People tend to exercise less in the winter than they do in the summer. The most common reason for cutting back on exercise is the dark, cold days. Those excuses are pretty good, right? Well, here's the problem. SAD sufferers mostly get SAD in the winter. With winter comes lack of energy, carbohydrate craving, and sadness. Those factors often result in weight gain that can then make SAD sufferers feel even worse about themselves and more sluggish. Exercise can increase energy, decrease cravings, and improve mood. Therefore, in this section we talk a little about exercising in the winter and a few of our favorite types of exercise activities.

Working out in winter

Do you head indoors in the winter? Many people do. But with a little preparation, winter workouts can continue outdoors, even when it's cold. Why bother? Because if you suffer from SAD, being outside, even for a short period of time, can decrease or even eliminate your symptoms.

When the weather is bad, protect yourself and still enjoy the great outdoors with these tips:

- ✔ **Dress warmly.** Wear layers of clothing. Make sure that the first layer draws moisture away from your body. Polypropylene is a synthetic, lightweight material that provides *wicking* (draws away moisture). Fleece is a good choice for the second layer. Fleece is comfortable, thin, and dries quickly. Cotton is a poor choice because it stays wet and gets too heavy. The third should keep the wind and water out but should be breathable. Synthetic materials that are tightly woven and waterproof make good choices. Many new fabrics and designs can keep you warm and cozy. Talk to a knowledgeable person at your local sporting goods or outdoor wear store.

- ✔ **Take special care of your head.** A majority of your body heat is lost through the head. So when you wear a hat, you retain that body heat. Wear a hat that covers your ears and consider wearing a scarf or another face covering, especially when it's really cold. Doing so can warm the air that you breathe and keep your face and lungs warm.

- ✔ **Wear mittens or gloves.** Mittens actually keep your hands warmer. But you may prefer gloves. When it's extremely cold, you can wear thin gloves inside your mittens. That way if you need to take your mittens off to do something, your hands remain protected.

- ✔ **Wear good shoes.** Whatever sport you're doing in the winter, make sure to wear the right kind of shoes. If your feet are uncomfortable, you're less likely to stay with your exercise. Cold or wet feet will send you inside. Consider insulated socks. Ask professional sportswear salespeople to help you pick out the right kind of gear.

- ✔ **Don't forget your sunscreen.** Although a little sun is good for you, sun reflected on snow can still give you a sunburn. Be sure to wear sunscreen and carry extra lip gloss or lip balm for comfort.

- ✔ **Wear reflective clothing.** If you're exercising when the light is dim, be extra careful and wear clothing with reflecting material so you can be seen by other people on the road.

- ✔ **Drink plenty of liquids.** Even winter activities can leave you sweaty and dehydrated. Water is probably the best choice, but coffee or tea can dehydrate you further.

Alcohol actually can interfere with your body's shivering mechanism and cause your body to lose heat quickly.

✔ **Go inside.** If you experience shortness of breath, pain, or numbness, go inside. If symptoms don't subside, seek medical care.

Pumping your heart and lungs

Aerobic exercise gets your heart beating and your blood circulating faster. *Aerobic* actually means *with oxygen,* and this type of exercise requires a lot of oxygen to carry it out. The benefits of aerobic exercise include

✔ Strengthening of the heart

✔ Toning muscles

✔ Strengthening and improving respiration

✔ Increased energy

✔ Better oxygenation

✔ High-impact activities can reduce bone loss

You have a lot of choices when it comes to aerobic exercise. You can ride a bike, jog, play tennis (singles is better than doubles), take an aerobic exercise class at a gym, play basketball, run, kick box, hike, swim, or walk briskly (enough to get you a bit out of breath), all of which can be done at almost any time of year.

In the winter you can ice skate, cross-country ski, snow shoe, and play ice hockey. Or if you're totally an extremist, you may try ice swimming. Ice fishing may be fun, but doesn't cut it as an aerobic sport unless there's a bunch of hiking to get there.

Building up muscles

Strength training is good for you to. This category of exercise is known as anaerobic. The advantages of anaerobic exercise include building muscle and burning calories. The calories part is especially useful to SAD sufferers who often struggle with weight gain.

You don't need those pricey, as-seen-on-TV weight machines. You don't even need to have a set of dumbbells. You can accomplish muscle building through multiple methods such as sit-ups, push-ups, lunges, or squats. For help with developing an exercise routine, take a look at *Fitness For Dummies,* 3rd Edition, by Suzanne Schlosberg and Liz Neporent (Wiley) and *Workouts For Dummies* by Tamilee Webb and Lori Seeger (Wiley).

Don't try to do too much anaerobic exercise in the beginning. You can end up with sore muscles or even cause a muscle strain or pull. Consider getting a personal trainer for the first few sessions and then consult with one once a month or so after that. It's not as expensive as you may think and could save you from injury as well as personalize your training.

Stretching and moving with yoga

Yoga has been around for a few years — about 5,000 or so. There are many different types of yoga; however, they all involve postures, breathing, and meditation. Yoga joins the body and the mind.

Yoga can be helpful for just about anyone. You don't have to be particularly limber or flexible to start. A well-trained yoga teacher can instruct you on taking care of your body and not push you into doing more than you can do. Yoga isn't a competitive sport.

Here are some of the most common forms:

- ✔ **Hatha yoga:** This choice is for the beginning yoga student. It's usually gentle and slow. You practice a variety of poses, which improve your balance and breathing and stretch your muscles. Hatha yoga is very relaxing.

- ✔ **Ashtanga yoga:** This form is also known as power yoga, and it helps you build endurance. You repeat certain poses quickly and get a challenging workout that makes you sweat! Check out *Power Yoga For Dummies* by Doug Swenson (Wiley).

- ✔ **Bikram yoga:** Prepare to sweat! This yoga, which is also called *Hot yoga,* is practiced in a room heated to about 100 degrees. The heat and sweating are supposed to cleanse your body and loosen up your muscles.

Check with your doctor before trying Bikram yoga. Don't try Bikram yoga if you have high blood pressure or cardiac problems. If your doctor gives you the go ahead, be sure to drink a lot of fluid (throughout your yoga session) to reduce the risk of dehydration.

- ✔ **Vinyasa yoga:** This type usually refers to a class that completes a series of poses called Sun Salutations. This type of yoga can be a little more aerobic than Hatha yoga but is less vigorous than Ashtanga.

- ✔ **Kundalini yoga:** This form involves more emphasis on breathing and energy (called prana). You perform rapid movement through a series of poses integrated with breathing and sometimes chanting.

For more information about yoga, check out *Yoga For Dummies* by Georg Feuerstein, Larry Payne, and Lilias Folan (Wiley).

Why bring up yoga in a book about SAD? Yoga has been shown to reduce stress and anxiety. It can be practiced in order to prevent or manage depression, including the seasonal kind. Try it, you just may like it.

Chapter 16

Feeling Good about Having Fun

. . . .

In This Chapter

▶ Realizing pleasure's power

▶ Deciding it's okay to feel good

▶ Picking positive, fun activities

▶ Having happy holidays

▶ Enjoying what life has already given you

. . . .

Seasonal affective disorder (SAD) steals your pleasure, saps energy, and feeds feelings of guilt. SAD sufferers, like those with any type of depression, feel blah and apathetic. Activities that once seemed enjoyable no longer hold the same appeal. The world looks bleak and devoid of delights. You may even feel like you don't deserve to feel good. If you feel this way now or during the colder months, don't buy into it! You deserve and need a little enjoyment just like everyone else.

Pleasure is more than just pleasurable — it's good for you! This chapter takes you further and encourages an exploration of pleasure. We look at the benefits of seeking and enjoying positive activities. Because the holidays are often an especially difficult time if you suffer from SAD, we also tell you how to brighten up winter celebrations. Finally, we discuss how appreciation can help you savor the pleasures you create for yourself.

This chapter isn't intended to fill your life with purpose and meaning while obliterating all traces of SAD. This chapter is designed simply to help you start the process of treating yourself a little better by giving a boost to your pleasurable pursuits.

Discovering the Power of Pleasure

What is pleasure? We'll start with the root word of pleasure, which is please. Add in pleasing and pleasant. If you look these words up in a dictionary or a thesaurus, you may encounter other words such as joy, satisfaction, good feelings, fun, enjoyable, and more. Pleasure is like a bright, sunny spring day with a clear sky, all the flowers in bloom, the trees bursting with green leaves, birds singing, bugs buzzing, and your allergies completely in check. What's more, you experience the day exactly as it is. Get the picture?

But if you're currently experiencing an episode of SAD, most of life's usual pleasures won't "appear" especially enjoyable to you. (We put the word "appear" in quotes because the appearance is a deceptive illusion created by your depressed mind.) Caught up in SAD, a day that really is sunny may seem dark. But your perception can be tuned more toward reality.

Scientists know that depression harms your health. In fact, the magnitude of depression's effects is at least as large as many other known health risk factors such as high cholesterol, smoking, and high blood pressure. Fortunately, pleasurable pursuits exert a positive influence on your health, emotions, and longevity.

If you push yourself to start trying what are known as healthy pleasures, you may indeed find them minimally enjoyable at first. But if you continue, you may inevitably discover that the joy starts returning. And as it does, the benefits of pleasure start mounting, and sunny days appear as sunny days!

These benefits go far beyond alleviating depressed moods. Hundreds of studies have now shown that pleasure and joy affect you in amazing ways:

- ✔ Substantially reduces risks of heart disease
- ✔ Reduces feelings of chronic pain
- ✔ Improves your immune system
- ✔ Adds years to your life
- ✔ Reduces the negative impact of stress

Feeling Good about Feeling Good

Especially when depressed, many people feel that they don't *deserve* to experience pleasure in their lives. More often than not, the parents of these folks instilled messages such as "You have to earn everything," "Having fun is a waste of time," "Work is the only honorable thing a person can do," or "Work equals worth." In other words, they've been taught that fun, pleasure, and entertainment are frivolous and that one should focus on nothing but accomplishments, success, and achieving goals.

In addition, such parents tend to criticize failures and mistakes, whether large or small. No wonder their children grow up believing that they don't deserve pleasure or happiness. Even if you had a great childhood with perfect parents, when you're under the influence of SAD, you're probably sending yourself pleasure-robbing messages. Whether you heard such messages as a child or are telling them to yourself, you can learn to overcome their effects on you.

Consider the following alternative perspectives:

- ✔ **Fun and pleasure recharge your batteries.** Even if you value work and accomplishing goals over pleasure and fun, please realize that studies show people do better and are more productive when they take time out to recharge.

- ✔ **Eliminating pleasures increases your risks for depression.** And depression reduces your productivity. Once again, the human system has a true need for reasonable amounts of pleasure.

- ✔ **Joy, play, and pleasure improve your health.** Regularly experiencing pleasure in your life literally improves your health.

- ✔ **People don't have to earn happiness.** Where is it written that you must accomplish three goals (or ten or 20 or whatever) before you can deserve to be happy? Is it possible that just because you're human, you can let yourself be happy? If you're not satisfied with your accomplishments, you can work on that too, but it will be easier if you first allow for a little joy in your life.

- ✔ **Talk back to the mind chatter.** If your depressed mind tells you that you don't deserve pleasure because you're a lazy person, you don't deserve to feel good, or some other similar drivel, develop answers to those thoughts. When you hear your negative thoughts trying to dissuade you from bringing pleasure back into your life, try repeating these statements:

    - I don't have to earn pleasure; it's a basic human right.

    - I can be imperfect and still have some fun in life.

    - Pleasure and happiness will make me healthier.

    - I don't have to listen to my parents' old messages about work and perfection.

If repeating the statements above over and over don't help you to start increasing the pleasures in your life, consider reading or rereading Chapters 9 and 10. The principles outlined in those chapters can be easily applied to the thoughts that may stand in the way of your pursuit of pleasure.

Choosing Positive Pleasures

Pleasure is one word with millions of meanings for different people. For instance, take our relative as an example. He enjoys being dropped out of a helicopter in freezing cold weather and hurling himself down a steep, dangerous mountain. He actually pays a lot of money for his kind of pleasurable activity —

helicopter skiing. We think it sounds like an extremely scary and unpleasant activity. We would never pay money to do something like that.

So, what sounds like cold, painful torture may be pleasurable to someone. Nevertheless, pleasure can be broken down into categories. Because we want you to explore pleasure in various venues, we now review your pleasure options.

Seeking sensations

The more usual form of sensory-based pleasures are those that simply bring positive feelings because they feel good, look good, taste good, sound good, or smell good.

You can get pleasure from many sources:

- A massage (one of our favorites)
- A warm sunny day
- Changing into a comfortable set of sweats after work
- Chocolate (the richer the better)
- Mozart (the Beatles, or even heavy metal)
- Petting a dog (our dogs vote for this one)
- Pizza
- Red wine (okay, white will do too)
- Rembrandt
- Sex
- The sight of sand and water stretching as far as you can see
- The smell of baking bread
- The sound of waves
- The touch of an ocean breeze
- Exercise (see Chapter 15)

The sensory pleasures are one category of pleasure that you can easily overdo. Thus, you don't want to overindulge in red wine, chocolate, and pizza. Ben Franklin had it right when he suggested the virtues of moderation and temperance.

On the other hand, too many people avoid sensory pleasures out of a feeling that they don't deserve them. See "Feeling Good about Feeling Good" earlier in this chapter if this issue applies to you.

Getting together

This category of pleasure involves being with someone or a group of people. Human beings are social animals. Research shows that people who connect well with others are healthier and happier than folks who don't.

Social pleasures include the following:

- Being with your partner
- Giving a talk
- Going to a party
- Playing with children
- Spending time with a neighbor
- Talking with a friend on the phone
- Talking with friends
- Text messaging (though we're too old to really get this one)
- Visiting a friend in a hospital or nursing home
- Visiting with family
- Having lunch with a friend
- Watching a baby sleep

Doing something helpful or nice for someone else can also increase your sense of well-being. Contribute to charity, shovel snow for a neighbor, or tutor a child. You can also clean out your closets and donate the results to a local homeless shelter. See Chapter 19 for more information about the value of contributing to others.

Learning and creativity

This pleasure category involves discovering something new, learning a skill, satisfying curiosity, inventing, creating, and finding out answers. Half of the fun lies in the quest. Allow your mind to roam. Consider the possibilities:

- Change the color scheme in your house
- Create a sculpture
- Draw a picture
- Learn to dance
- Plant a flower

- ✔ Read a good book
- ✔ Reorganize your home office
- ✔ Research a topic of interest (you don't have to do anything with the results)
- ✔ Search for new works of art or crafts for your home
- ✔ Sow a vegetable garden
- ✔ Take a continuing education class
- ✔ Take an art lesson
- ✔ Write a poem or letter

Fact is, anything new or interesting can bring you pleasure. For example, we're taking Spanish lessons. Why? For no particular reason other than the mental stimulation and the joy of learning. *Queremos estudiar algo nuevo* (translation: We like to study something new). In fact, after a study session, we can feel our brains buzz with intrigue.

Laughing and playing

Laughter really is the best medicine and helps you stay healthy and happy. It can reduce pain by releasing endorphins that also improve moods. You can also burn calories by laughing and exercise your face and abdominal muscles.

Find humor in everyday life. Laugh a little at yourself. Visit a playground and watch children laughing. You can go to a comedy club, read a funny book, watch comedies on television or at the movies, or share a joke with a friend. Just laugh.

And don't be shy about joining in on the fun you find. A fabulous way to have a great time is to play with kids. If you don't have any children of your own, go hang out with friends who do.

Get together with friends and play. You can go bowling (a sport with resurging popularity), go to a ballgame, or play a board game. Start a poker night. Just play.

Succeeding in small steps

People are pleased when they're successful. The challenge of mastering a skill, doing something well, achieving personal success, figuring out how to program the new television, or finishing a project can be rewarding and positive.

One way to achieve success is to set modest goals. By modest we mean something significantly smaller than launching a new business. Take small steps. Set goals you know you can meet in a short period of time. For example, make your goal that of increasing your savings account by a small amount each month instead of focusing on amassing a million dollars over the next 15 years. Or set your goal at 15 minutes of exercise five times a week with the intention to gradually build it up from there, as opposed to setting an ambitious goal of an hour per day right from the start.

You can maximize feelings of success and accomplishment by writing down your goals and tracking your progress. Keep track on your calendar or tape a chart or list on your refrigerator. The format of your tracking doesn't matter, but doing it helps you stay focused on your goals and aware of your successes. If your tracking shows some slips along the way, use that information to get yourself going again instead of beating yourself up.

Success and achieving goals can result in much satisfaction for most people. However, if you're a perfectionist and deride yourself unmercifully whenever you make the smallest mistake, you should probably minimize your use of "success" as your route to increasing pleasure. Try our other suggestions in this chapter first. We also recommend that you read the earlier section, "Feeling Good about Feeling Good" as well as Chapters 9 and 10 before tackling "success" as your means of finding pleasure.

Traveling and taking breaks

Travel and vacations include most of the pleasures listed in this chapter such as creativity, learning, social, and sensory delights. In addition, travel and vacations provide a crucial time for rejuvenating and resting. And if you have SAD, travel toward the sunshine makes a lot of sense. See Chapter 14 for more hints about travel.

You don't have to have a ton of money to go on vacation. You can take vacations at home. Stock up on food that's easy to prepare, rent some movies, or schedule a few hot baths or massages. As long as you make time for rest and recreation, it will be a vacation.

Take an inventory of your life. What activities are you doing in the next week that bring you pleasure? You don't have to engage in big projects, have huge parties, or take big vacations to have fun. Find a way to get pleasure out of the small things in life.

Illuminating Celebrations

Throughout recorded history, civilizations have consistently developed celebrations around the time of the winter solstice (the shortest day of the year). This day also of course represents the demarcation of when the light begins to return and lengthen each day; in other words, the rebirth of hope for many people. Most of these celebrations involve light.

Whatever traditions you celebrate (and even if you don't celebrate any), we encourage you to brighten up your home and your world at this time of year. Consider the following bright ideas:

- ✔ **Build more fires.** Fires are cozy, festive, romantic, and add warmth. Sitting by a fire brings people together. Check out three popular options for creating festive fires:

    - **Fire pits:** You can buy pits or dig one in your backyard. Fire pits come in all shapes, sizes, and prices. You can buy simple metal containers or elaborate stone and copper pieces of art.

    - **Fireplaces:** If you have one, start using it more often. We like wood, but some people prefer the ease and clean burn of gas logs. Remember to maintain the safety of your fireplace — have your chimney cleaned per manufacturer recommendations.

    - **Wood or pellet stoves:** If you don't already have a fireplace, many people enjoy woodstoves, and they can be made to fit into most homes.

    Never leave a fire unattended. Make sure you use a safe container. And every house should have a working fire extinguisher and smoke detectors.

- ✔ **Burn candles.** Candles are as much a part of the holidays as festive foods. They come in endless shapes, styles, smells, and colors. You can never have too many candles. Although they can hardly serve as light therapy (see Chapter 5), they do brighten the environment and your spirits.

    Keep lit candles out of the way of children and pets. Candles can be hazardous if not watched — they account for almost 5 percent of home fires in the United States. Always use a candle holder and don't allow them to burn all the way down.

✔ **Put out more light bulbs.** Again, this approach can't completely substitute for light therapy, but you can increase your exposure to lumens (see Chapter 5) by adding more lamps, light fixtures, and decorative strings of lights.

Consider using lower energy consuming bulbs that also happen to last much longer than traditional incandescent light bulbs. New light emitting diode (LED) lights are available, as are fluorescent bulbs that fit standard sockets.

Appreciating What You Have

However, as you start your pleasure seeking, it's also important for you to notice and appreciate your endeavors. So many people blitz through their lives, bouncing from one experience after another, and yet they fail to savor what they're doing. They always look toward the *next* thing they want to do while neglecting what they're doing now. If that process describes you, stop now! Take a moment to see, feel, taste, smell, and truly relish each experience in the now.

A good way to start appreciating the small pleasures in life is to track them. Then take a few moments to describe each one. You don't have to spend a lot of time on this task; simply jot down a few descriptive words and *notice* your experiences. Start out by trying to record at least four positive experiences each day.

Check out Bob's story and his example in Table 16-1:

Bob finally gets out of bed at 6:30 a.m. after tossing and turning for the past hour. He leaves for a business trip tomorrow and is already ruminating about all that he has to do to get ready. As usual, too many details are left until the last moment, and he feels pressured to do them all.

It's cold and cloudy this Monday morning. He trudges outside to get the newspaper, and the wind starts to pick up. At least he's going to California tomorrow where the weather will probably be better. Bob's two dogs wait at the front door when he gets in with the paper. They greet him as if he had been gone for hours instead of seconds. Looking down at them dancing at his feet, leaping into the air, Bob can't help but smile. He realizes that he's let himself get down again, thinking about the past (not getting things done) and the future (too many things to do).

Bob's dogs' joy inspires him to write down a few things that he's feeling positive about right now.

Table 16-1	Bob's Positive Experiences	
Day	*Experience*	*Thoughts, Feelings, and Sensations*
Monday	My dogs jumping and wagging their tails	Smiling, feeling lucky to have the dogs in my life; they remind me about simple pleasures.
	Sitting for a few minutes with coffee and the newspaper	I'm lucky to have this time. The coffee tastes good.
	My wife trying to help me out of my bad mood this morning	I appreciate her. I'm lucky to have someone at home who's supportive.
	My job	Even though it gets too busy, it's a pretty good job for me. I like the work, and the travel can be fun at times.
	My home	I love living where I do. Even when the weather is bad, it's beautiful and peaceful.

Bob takes a few minutes to jot down the positive parts of his morning. It doesn't take long for his mood to improve. He knows that his tendency to become overstressed about travel has a long history. However, he can easily turn it around by counting his blessings and appreciating the small pleasures in his life.

Part V
Life after SAD

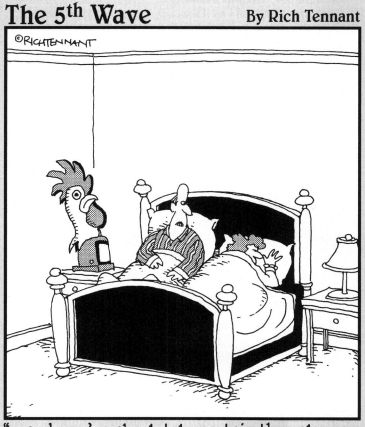

"...and you're absolutely certain the salesman said this dawn simulator only regulates the morning light and nothing more?"

In this part . . .

Seasonal affective disorder (SAD) comes and goes when left untreated. You can also have a relapse after being successfully treated. In this part, you begin to understand your risk of relapse, what to look out for, and what you can do to minimize relapse. You also find out how to use mindful acceptance to reduce relapse. Finally, you discover how to find a more meaningful, fulfilling life after SAD.

Chapter 17

Reducing the Risk of Relapse

$\bullet \bullet$

In This Chapter

▶ Stopping SAD before it starts

▶ Recognizing SAD event triggers

▶ Turning SAD thoughts around

▶ Stomping out SAD relapse

$\bullet \bullet$

Seasonal affective disorder (SAD) is, by definition, a problem related to the seasons. And the conditions that start SAD — the darkening days of winter — repeat themselves every season. So, it comes as no surprise that the relapse risk of SAD is very high.

As you delve into this chapter, you look beyond recovery to the looming risk of relapse. SAD symptoms can begin quietly and catch you unaware. We tell you about your risk and what you should look out for.

Heading Off a SAD Relapse

Depending on where you live, preparations for winter can be as simple as pulling some sweaters down from the top shelf in your closet or as complicated as conducting a thorough energy audit of your home. In places where SAD tends to hit most often, winter preparation presents a daunting challenge. In some climates there are snow blowers to tune up, numerous cords of wood to chop, windows and doorways to seal, and extensive wardrobes to changeover.

Wherever you live, our advice is to plan ahead; don't wait until the first big snowstorm hits. Your energy and motivation are likely better in late summer and early fall than by November. If you wait, you may just feel totally overwhelmed by the winter months. So make your list and check it twice.

Consider these items for your preparations:

✔ **Prepare and repair your vehicles.** Put winter-weight oil in your cars if required in your area. Make sure your tires are good and decide if you need snow tires. If your car hasn't been tuned up, do it before winter hits and have the battery checked too.

✔ **Purchase snow and ice equipment early.** Maybe you don't need a snow blower, but if you do, make sure it's tuned up. Buy snow shovels before it snows! Our last snow in New Mexico (we had an all-time record of 19 inches in contrast to our usual 2 inches) caused a run on hardware stores where snow shovels and rock salt became as scarce as bikinis in Fairbanks, Alaska, in December.

✔ **Make sure your furnace and fireplace are ready.** Check the air filter and clean it. If your furnace runs on propane, fill up the tank. If you burn wood, have the chimney cleaned and stock up on wood early whether you chop your own or buy it.

✔ **Review your winter wardrobe.** Dig out those gloves, scarves, sweaters, hats, and heavy coats. Check their condition and replace and/or clean as needed. When you purchase new outdoor wear, go for warmth over style.

✔ **Brighten up your house.** Even if you decide not to use a bright light therapy lamp, look for ways to increase light in your house. Consider putting out festive candles. See Chapter 5 for more ideas on how to brighten your house.

✔ **Shop early.** If you're someone who celebrates the holiday season with gifts, buy them early, before you have any loss of energy and enthusiasm.

Ideally, the best way to deal with relapse is to prevent it from happening in the first place. Of course that's not always possible, but you can do many things to improve your odds. If you've gone three or more winters without a recurrence of SAD or winter blues, you may not need to put as much effort into prevention. But if your last episode of SAD has occurred more recently than that, consider implementing the ideas in this section.

What else can you do to be prepared? In addition to taking steps to prepare your home, wardrobe, and car for the winter months, you may want to get a tune up for your mind and body. Take care of dental work, get eyes checked, see your doctor, visit your therapist, and enlist and educate a friend to keep an eye on you. Consider joining a gym and having a consultation with one of its personal trainers. The better shape you are in, the better you'll do through the winter months. Get the momentum started *before* the dark days come on.

You can also reduce stress and simplify your life. People with SAD often report feeling down in the winter even when they don't have full-blown episodes. Energy and motivation are at a low. So, as much as you can, avoid overloading your calendar, don't volunteer for huge projects, and leave cleaning the garage for the spring or get it done in early fall. See Chapter 12 for more ideas on letting go and getting help.

Finally, plan for some fun and meaningful activities. Make sure that you take good care of yourself. You can better handle some sadness if you take time to do what gives you pleasure and a sense of fulfillment. Please refer to Chapters 15 and 19 for more ideas.

Recognizing Relapse Trigger Events

Certain risk factors make SAD relapse more likely, and you can't always avoid these difficult events. However, knowing the events that can trigger a SAD relapse can help you be on guard against letting SAD sneak in. But be on the lookout and watch out for times when

- ✔ **You're physically sick or injured.** Illness and injury often lead to depression. The stress taxes your physical and emotional resources. SAD takes advantage of this weakness to reappear. Therefore, you should be especially kind to yourself when your body's hurting.

  Major heart problems are a particularly high-risk issue for depression in general. So it makes sense that (formal studies haven't been conducted) they also pose a risk for SAD relapse. Anytime you're in the hospital, your sleep schedule gets disturbed. So illness and hospitalization combine to increase your risks.

- ✔ **You suffer a loss.** When a loved one leaves, through death or other separation, you have a greater risk of getting ill or relapsing into depression. Loss of money, status, or a role (such as children leaving home or retirement) can also increase risk. Depression on top of loss makes recovery all the more difficult. If you previously suffered from SAD and experience personal loss, consider working through strategies in this chapter.

- ✔ **You're not getting enough sleep.** SAD symptoms can get worse when you aren't rested. Even if your SAD has remitted, your risk of relapse increases when tired. Of course for most people, one of the symptoms of SAD is chronic fatigue. So, poor sleep can be the start of a vicious cycle (see Chapter 13 on how to get your ZZZs).

✔ **You experience a big change in your life.** Even positive changes such as getting married, having a baby, or getting a promotion cause stress. Excitement about the change can trigger fears and worries that spin into a relapse of SAD symptoms. Whenever significant changes occur, be scanning for SAD.

✔ **Your close relationship is in trouble.** Relationships usually provide important, helpful support and even buffer against depression. Studies have shown that people who are in a committed relationship are generally happier than other folks (when things are going well). But when an important relationship experiences conflict, it can pose a risk for a new episode of SAD.

Defusing stressful events

Bad things happen. Fires, floods, hurricanes, tornadoes, and terrorism are adverse events that may occur in your life. So you should have an emergency survival kit. Box up supplies: first-aid, water, food, extra medication, batteries, blankets, and portable radios.

You can be prepared and fully aware, but if everything seems to be going swimmingly, it may be difficult to see the triggers (that can sometimes be like landmines) and without warning SAD can reappear. Other life events can also throw you off track. This unexpected relapse of SAD happened to Christopher when he experienced several major life changes, got a cold, and felt exhausted.

> **Christopher** cheerfully wraps another glass in newspaper and places it into the cardboard box. He looks forward to the move from an apartment into his first new home. He and his wife expect their first child to be born in a few months, and he can't recall a time in his life that he was happier. Everything he's dreamed of seems to be coming true. Even the cold he's been fighting can't get him down.
>
> He recalls the last few years in college when he had recurrent depressive episodes. The doctor he saw diagnosed him with SAD. Now, he looks outside at the winter snow and believes that the diagnosis was made in error. The winter sun sets early in northern Maine, but this year, Christopher remains chipper.
>
> The move takes many hours and Christopher falls into bed well after midnight and totally exhausted. His coughing wakes him up too early in the new house. He feels momentarily disoriented. He looks over at his sleeping wife and thinks, "What have I done? I can't believe we bought this house. What if we lose our jobs? How am I going to support my family? We'll go broke making these mortgage payments."
>
> Christopher feels a knot of worry tighten in his stomach. He gets out of bed and heads for the kitchen. He grabs last night's cold pizza from the

refrigerator and quickly eats the three leftover pieces. Not feeling satisfied, he hunts through unpacked boxes for something else to eat. He finds a box of stale cheese crackers and eats mindlessly while continuing to worry. His wife finds him sitting glumly among cracker crumbs and cold pizza crusts. SAD has returned to Christopher's life. It hit him before he knew what was happening, and he hadn't been prepared for the blow.

Christopher's story illuminates how risk factors can contribute to a SAD relapse. Christopher faced big changes in his life with a new house and baby on the way. In addition, he was tired from the move as well as fighting a cold. These risk factors plus the usual risk of decreased sunlight in the winter pushed him into a SAD relapse. We don't want SAD to re-emerge in your life. Fortunately, there are things you can do to prepare.

Being prepared

To try to prepare for the unexpected in your life, you should first make a list of all the things you fear happening to you (rejection, being fired, conflict at work, and so on) at some point in the future. Then answer the following questions for each of those events *before* they even happen. In addition, you can consult these questions and review them when unexpected trouble hits.

- ✔ How much meaning will this event have for me in one year?
- ✔ Have I (or someone I know) ever successfully dealt with something like this before?
- ✔ Is this happening as bad as I'm making it out to be?
- ✔ What advice would I give a friend of mine for dealing with something like this?
- ✔ Is there a way for me to grow from this occurrence?

The story of Isabella demonstrates how even big challenges can be plowed through successfully by using our list of questions for getting through tough times. She uses the questions after a serious car crash because she worries about a relapse of her SAD from previous winters.

> **Isabella** taps the brakes lightly as she approaches the on ramp to the freeway. The snow melted during the day, but the evening brings lower temperatures, and the slush is beginning to freeze. She glides onto the freeway without skidding. But suddenly, immediately in front of her, brake lights flash. Reacting quickly, Isabella stomps on her brakes, and loses control of her car, which spins out of her lane, then is hit by another vehicle. Her car crashes against the guardrail. Isabella screams as the air bags inflate. She breathes hard and panics to get untangled from her car. Someone helps her. Traffic has stopped. Sirens scream in the distance. Isabella shakes from fear, but seems to be unhurt. Her car is totaled.

In the following days she deals with the police, the insurance company, and the rental car agency. She feels lucky to be alive, but the stress has sent her mood spiraling down. She was proud to have gotten through the first part of winter without a relapse of SAD, but worries now that she may be heading there. She answers the following questions to help her defend against a recurrence of her SAD.

- How much meaning will this event have for me in one year?

  In a year, I'll still think about this accident once in a while and probably be relieved that I wasn't hurt.

- Have I (or someone I know) ever successfully dealt with something like this before?

  Not really. But as much as I hate all the hassles, I'm managing the details pretty well. Furthermore, I do know other people who've had this happen, and I know how they handled it.

- Is this happening as bad as I'm making it out to be?

  I was so scared when it happened. I still can't believe that I didn't get hurt. My car was totaled, and that's pretty awful, but again, I guess it could've been worse.

- What advice would I give a friend of mine for dealing with something like this?

  I would tell my friend to be thankful for having insurance, a seat belt, and an air bag!

- Is there a way for me to grow from this occurrence?

  My biggest challenge will be to drive again when the conditions are icy. I know that people say to get back on the horse when you fall off. This task will be hard; I may avoid the freeways when it's icy. I am pretty proud of myself for not completely falling apart. Maybe I can handle the bad stuff when it happens. That's good to know.

Isabella discovered that these questions helped her by decreasing her negative thinking. She certainly didn't think the accident was a good thing, but she figured out that she was able to cope. In fact, by discovering she had more strength than she had thought, she actually grew from the experience and felt more resilient than ever.

Accept the inevitable challenges of life. When difficult times, unexpected hassles, or unavoidable accidents happen, try to adapt, grow, and cope. If you find that you need more support, reach out and ask for help from others. Seek counsel from a trusted friend, family member, or get professional help. Being strong also involves knowing when you can't go it alone.

Recognizing SAD-Prone Thinking

Thinking is a key trigger for SAD. Two types of thinking pose a risk for relapse with SAD. The first type is *negative* thinking (see Chapters 9 and 10 for more information about negative thinking). Negative thinking sounds like this:

- ✔ I can't stand it when it's cold outside.
- ✔ I hate the winter.
- ✔ When the sun sets early, I don't want to go anywhere.
- ✔ I'm never happy when it's cold.
- ✔ I can't be productive in the winter.

So, if you notice negative thoughts running through your mind, even if you're not feeling depressed yet, you may run a high risk of encountering a SAD episode.

If you do notice negative thinking, don't beat yourself up. That's called having negative thoughts about your negative thoughts. Such self-ridicule can easily spiral into a whirlpool of negativity and depression. Instead, work through the ideas in this chapter in sections "Heading Off a SAD Relapse" and "Dealing with Relapse".

Being overly optimistic

A second type of thinking can also increase your chances of relapse. This one just may surprise you. If you have *excessively* optimistic, *overly* positive thoughts, you actually run a relapse risk!

How can that be? If you read Chapters 9 and 10, you know that we tell you to think positively. So now you're probably thinking we're a little crazy. But if you practice cognitive therapy, you know that it attempts to help you find distortions in your thinking and develop realistic perspectives of yourself and the world. So, the following are examples of *overly positive* thoughts that could set you up for trouble:

- ✔ I have no doubt that I have conquered my SAD forever.
- ✔ I can handle anything now.
- ✔ I have complete, total control of my moods now.

✔ Nothing could ever upset me now that I've mastered the skills presented in this book.

✔ Winter could never get me down again.

Why do we say these thoughts are too positive? Because they simply aren't realistic. You have a very good chance of conquering your SAD, and you may very well be able to avoid a relapse, but it's far from a certainty. When expectations are set too high, they're easily punctured by reality. You can't control your moods 100 percent of the time. Take Judy for example:

> **Judy** is the CEO of a small corporation and suffered from three episodes of SAD in the past. However, she got treatment with cognitive therapy and medication and now feels terrific. She's absolutely certain that her depressed days are behind her.
>
> Judy spends time in a chat room with fellow SAD sufferers. She lets the chat room members know about her wonderful experience with cognitive therapy. She tells them that she's conquered any and all negative thoughts that may come her way. She writes that winter is her favorite season now, and she's positive that she'll never have another relapse. A number of the other members talk about their relapses, and Judy finds it difficult to connect with them. She drops out of the group, no longer feeling a need for their support.
>
> A couple of weeks later, Judy's Board of Directors decides to reduce her anticipated bonus this year because the company has not done quite as well as they'd hoped. Judy feels stunned and angry — so much so that she fails to use her skills for dealing with difficult events that she'd acquired from her therapist. She faces January in a foul mood that deepens into depression as the dark days continue.

Cognitive therapy helps prevent SAD relapse. However, you want to temper such optimism like Judy's with the realistic knowledge that bad things do happen. Judy fell further into her depression that she may have otherwise avoided because she was overly optimistic about her recovery.

Bringing thoughts into balance

Optimism and hope are good things, and we want you to have them! At the same time, realizing that you need to prepare for unpleasant or unexpected events helps you deal with them better when and if they occur. Balance is key — moderation works best. So if you find your head filled with any words that are black and white or all or none, step back and rethink a little. Other signs of extreme thinking (whether negative or positive) are words like "always," and "never." When you hear yourself thinking in extremes, try to consider using moderate thinking such as "sometimes," "usually," "often," and so on.

In the preceding example, Judy believed so completely that she could *never* experience a relapse that she became vulnerable to the negative event of having her bonus reduced. Had she instead realized that relapse is always a risk and prepared for the eventuality of life's negative encounters, she probably would have coped better.

Dealing with Relapse

SAD has a stealthy nature. Sometimes even the best preparation leaves a gap, and you can slowly slip into a full-blown episode of SAD. The fact that the slip is gradual is useful because it gives you the opportunity to stop the slide before it gets too slippery to stop. Fortunately, there are signs that can tip you off to that slippery slope. Sometimes a trusted friend can help you stay alert to these signs.

Here are some of the most common early warning signs:

- ✔ **Snacking a little more than usual:** Prior to developing the intense carbohydrate cravings common to SAD, you may often report feeling hungry more between meals. You nibble a little more frequently and have a sense of emptiness in your stomach that wants to be filled. See Chapter 7 for a variety of ways to deal with this issue.

- ✔ **Creeping fatigue:** With full-blown SAD, tiredness can feel overpowering and drain all the energy out of your mind and body. Prior to that, you may find yourself hitting the snooze button a few more times than usual and just not feel like getting out of bed. You drag yourself out anyway, but may start procrastinating tasks a little more often. Chapters 13 and 15 give you ways for dealing with this early symptom.

- ✔ **Loss of enthusiasm:** Loss of enthusiasm precedes a more complete loss of pleasure and interest in things common to SAD. So be on the lookout for saying no to going out with friends or not laughing as much at work. These signs can be early issues that you need to address. Check out Chapters 14 and 16 for information about handling a loss of enthusiasm.

- ✔ **Growing irritability:** Usually you're fairly easy going, but when SAD starts up, the guy in the next lane cutting in front of you sets off a string of ugly words. You notice the small stuff is getting you sweaty. Irritability is often a symptom of depression. See Chapter 11 for tips on calming down.

- ✔ **Pessimistic thinking:** Cloudy dark thoughts can signal the beginning of SAD. You may find yourself believing that bad things happen and that you have very little control over outcomes. Check out Chapter 10 for a tune up for your thinking.

Getting some satisfaction

When SAD or depression are creeping up on you, often the first sign shows up in the form of deriving less pleasure or satisfaction from what you do as opposed to suddenly feeling overwhelming sadness. A declining sense of satisfaction often leads to other early symptoms such as sleeping and eating more. Those symptoms in turn can deepen into despair and full-blown SAD. Therefore, catching the early indications of reduced pleasure or satisfaction can help prevent relapse.

Instead of waiting for horribly depressing, difficult events and feelings to emerge, be on the lookout for anytime you sense that your thoughts may be cutting off the amount of satisfaction you normally expect from a previously enjoyed activity. You see what we mean in our example of Esperanza:

> **Esperanza** was diagnosed with SAD about three years ago, after she'd been depressed for winter after winter. As part of her recovery, her therapist suggested that she find an active hobby. She chose flamenco and ballroom dance. Today Esperanza loves to dance. She dances at least three times a week. She has talent and many admirers of her dancing.
>
> She did very well in her treatment and hasn't seen her therapist in two years. Lately, Esperanza has noticed just a slight drop in her usual feelings of satisfaction. She certainly isn't depressed, but she remembers what her therapist told her about early warning sides of SAD. She completes the SAD Thought Tracker and Evidence Based Thoughts Form in Table 17-1.

Here's how to use the forms followed by Esperanza's example:

✔ **Feelings and sensations:** In the first column, write down both your body's sensations and a feeling word that describes those sensations. Also rate the feeling words for intensity from 1 (very mild) to 100 (extremely intense or severe). Remember, the feeling doesn't have to be especially negative, it can be a mere subtle departure from the satisfaction you may normally experience.

✔ **Events:** In the second column, write down what you think may have triggered the feelings and sensations. Ask yourself what was going on.

✔ **Thoughts:** In the third column, record your thoughts about the event. Thoughts reflect the meaning or interpretation you have about what happened.

✔ **Evidence-Based Thoughts:** The fourth column is where you list your new, revised (evidence based) thoughts. You come up with those new thoughts by answering the following questions. They help you examine your initial thoughts and come up with a more balanced way of looking at what happened:

- What evidence do I have that either supports or refutes this thought?

- Do I have experiences in my life that can contradict this thought?

- Is this satisfaction interrupting thought distorted and can I come up with a more accurate, reasonable replacement thought?

✔ **Rating the Results:** Take another look at your feelings and indicate whether they've changed. Express what you feel you got from the exercise.

Table 17-1	SAD Thought Tracker and Evidence Based Thoughts Form		
Feelings and Sensations	*Events*	*Thoughts or Interpretations*	*Evidence-Based Thoughts*
I felt okay, but a little disappointed (30).	I won the dance contest.	I should've done better; I missed a step.	Everyone misses a step here and there. I need to watch out for my self-critic and tell her to shut up!
A little irritated (25).	Brandon said I looked beautiful.	He doesn't really mean it; he says that to everyone.	He doesn't really say that to everybody. Sometimes I need to just accept compliments for what they are.
Irritated, tense, and tired (35).	The parking lot was buried in snow, and I barely found a spot.	Maybe I should quit dance in the winter; it's just a hassle.	Sure it's a hassle, but I always enjoy myself when I get there. And dance is probably at least half of why I don't get SAD anymore. I don't want to listen to that kind of thought.

Rating the Results

Wow, I can see how those thoughts can sneak up on me and steal my satisfaction. It feels really good to catch them, and I can review some of the materials in other chapters of *Seasonal Affective Disorder For Dummies*. I'm glad I did this exercise.

Negative thinking can interrupt your satisfaction and happiness in a variety of subtle, but nefarious ways. You need to be on the lookout for such thoughts and catch them before they drag you under.

Doing what worked before

When you're depressed, you probably lack hope and motivation. You may even find yourself saying, "Why bother? I've tried other things before and they obviously didn't work — after all, I'm depressed again."

Ah, but that's just SAD thinking trying to control you. The good news actually is that anything that worked for you before is likely to work again. Just because you're in another episode doesn't mean that a new round of what you'd had success with in the past won't work now — quite the contrary, it probably will. Try out these options:

- ✔ **Behavior therapy:** If you managed your SAD symptoms by increasing pleasurable activities, exercise, or other strategies that involved changing what you do — do it again. You can benefit from reviewing the ideas in Chapters 14, 15, and 16.

- ✔ **Cognitive therapy:** Some of our clients come in for "booster" sessions — times for a tune up of their thinking. A few sessions are usually all it takes. You can go for these booster sessions before symptoms start or at the first warning sign. See Chapters 9 and 10 for more on cognitive therapy.

- ✔ **Light therapy:** If light therapy brightened up your mood before, then by all means, turn on the lights. Studies say that you likely need about the same time and intensity as you did during your last depression. The only way light therapy can prevent a relapse is if you use it before you detect symptoms of SAD flaring up. Review the nuts and bolts of using light therapy in Chapter 5.

- ✔ **Medication:** Some people prefer to start taking medication in the fall before symptoms start. See Chapter 6 for more about deciding to take medication for SAD.

- ✔ **Alternative treatments:** Perhaps you improved with other treatments such as melatonin, massage, acupuncture, or meditation. If so, resume these therapies. See Chapter 8 for more information on alternative treatments.

SAD relapse isn't uncommon. However, SAD symptoms can also mimic another problem or illness. Check with your healthcare provider to rule out any other medical conditions before treating your SAD on your own.

Trying something new

A relapse may occur at a time in your life that you aren't willing or able to resume what worked for you before. Maybe you want to get pregnant and avoid medication. Possibly you have responsibilities that make sitting in front of a light for 30 minutes a day too time consuming. Or perhaps you've tried the treatment that worked before, and it doesn't seem to be working to decrease your SAD symptoms.

The more strategies you have in your SAD arsenal, the better chance you have of defeating SAD. So, try something else if SAD returns. If you've been successful with light therapy, maybe try medication. Instead of taking medication, you may consider light therapy.

Try the cognitive therapy techniques outlined in Chapters 9 and 10. Studies find that people who've completed cognitive therapy are less likely to relapse. That's because the skills you acquire in this therapy change the way you think and help defend against negative thoughts. Consider contacting a mental health professional that uses cognitive-behavioral techniques. A therapist can be a supportive, kind coach for your journey back to health.

Chapter 18

Accepting Reasonable Sadness

*W*ait a minute here; isn't the pursuit of happiness considered an inalienable right? Heck, it's even written as such in the United States Declaration of Independence. Many people seek happiness relentlessly throughout their lives. And in spite of this zealous pursuit, evidence states that there's less happiness and more depression today than there was 50 years ago — even though there's more time and money available for this quest than ever before.

In part, that's because the pursuit of happiness is another paradox. The more you strive, push, and toil for achieving happiness, the more you absolutely *must have* happiness, and the less likely you are to find it. It's kind of like trying to grasp water in your fist.

But there's another way of getting there. Happiness will find *you* if you focus on living life fully, accept that there will be some sadness in your life, let go of being judgmental, retune your mind chatter, keep your esteem in balance, and take some time to be still. In a sense, happiness sneaks in the back door, but only if you immerse yourself in experiencing life in the present. The sections in this chapter tell you more about how to accomplish these goals.

Embracing Sadness

Everyone experiences sadness from time to time. Normal sadness is what happens when you experience losses, setbacks, and frustrations. When you're sad, your mood, zest, and energy decline for a day or two, but they usually improve with a little time. Depression and seasonal affective disorder

(SAD) are more than normal reactions to unpleasant events. These disorders last longer and dig in more deeply. See Chapter 2 for more information about the differences between sadness, grief, and depression and Chapter 19 for how to pull out of a bad mood.

However, if you feel that you can't stand the experience of "normal sadness," your bad feelings are actually likely to increase. Instead, wrap your arms around sadness, hug unhappiness, and squeeze your sorrow. Hold on; the point of a self-help book is to help you feel better, right? You may be thinking that we're now recommending that you just give up and be sad. That's not it at all.

Take this scenario for example: You blush easily, and you hate that you blush so easily. You're constantly worried about being embarrassed or upset. When people who hate blushing do blush, they likely think to themselves "This is terrible!" or "I look like an idiot!" or "Everyone's looking at me!"

Well, guess what? When you hate blushing, and getting red makes you miserable, you're more likely to blush. That's because the smallest incident raises your concern, and you react. A clumsy trip that goes unnoticed by most people becomes a major goof, and your face flushes. A mispronounced word, a careless error, a simple mistake takes on more significance because of the fear of blushing. The fear and embarrassment of blushing actually increase your risk. So, if you can accept your blushing tendencies, you're more likely *not* to blush.

The same principle holds true for SAD. When you can't stand to feel sad (or anxious or sleepy or embarrassed or whatever) then you're more likely to have those feelings. When your mind is on high alert for any sign of sadness, then you become extremely sensitive to the slightest bump.

The fact of the matter is that bad feelings are a part of life. But when you've suffered from SAD or depression, you can easily develop fear of negative feelings. So you constantly scan for any signs of bad moods. And when a bad mood does hit, you start saying things to yourself like:

- ✔ I just know that I'm slipping into a dark depression.
- ✔ I can't stand feeling depressed.
- ✔ I have no control over these horrible feelings.
- ✔ I'm hopeless.

So embracing sadness actually means that you *accept* some bad feelings as a part of life. It's actually a little paradoxical. The more you can accept a few bad feelings, the less bad feelings are likely to overtake you. When distress does occur, it seems more manageable. And you won't become depressed over a little sadness.

Acceptance represents a balance between working on negative thoughts, feelings, and behaviors and realizing that a certain degree of distressing emotions and thoughts exist in everyone's life.

Releasing Your Judgments

Listen to your thoughts. If you're like most people, you may notice instances of judging and evaluating yourself, others, experiences, and your environment. A majority of those judgments are likely pretty innocent. Examples of fairly harmless judgments include

- ✔ It's too hot in here.
- ✔ I don't like that dress she's wearing.
- ✔ That lecture was dull.
- ✔ The mall was too crowded today.
- ✔ I feel a little bloated today; my pants are too tight.

Those statements are judgments to be sure. However, you may not get too worked up about them either. On the other hand, making judgments can lead to distressing emotions such as anger, rage, irritability, sadness, being upset, melancholy, anxiety, and feeling helpless. In fact, the difference between the two types of judgments can be subtle. For example:

- ✔ I can't stand the unbearable heat in this room; I'm going to die.
- ✔ Her dress is horrible; she looks awful.
- ✔ That guy is an idiot; I couldn't stand listening to him.
- ✔ Every parking space was taken today. I hate crowds.
- ✔ I'm so fat that no one could like me.

The second list of judgments evokes the most emotions. Going from mild to painful judgments happens easily, so practice *non*-judgment. *Non-judgmental* thinking observes and describes without using highly critical adjectives and adverbs. Non-judgmental thinking takes an objective, detached stance. Mindfulness and non-judgmental thinking keeps you focused on present moments, experiences, and sensations.

Start the process by noticing when you use highly charged adjectives such as horrific, unbearable, wrong, disgusting, heinous, insufferable, and intolerable. Such words embellish novels nicely. However, they stir up emotions — that's good for a novel; bad when you think about what's going on in your life.

Non-judgmental conversation is how a meteorologist observes and talks about the weather: "A powerful storm system is moving across the eastern plains and may bring as much as 12 inches of snow." Contrast that style with the more attention-grabbing approach of a weather reporter on the 10 o'clock news: "This history-making storm front could bring howling winds, driving snow, and chaos. The snow will likely paralyze the city, snarl traffic, and cause horrific delays. Stay home and stay tuned for the developing crisis."

Because SAD is related to changes in both light and weather, we use the following example to show you the difference between a judgmental evaluative style and a mindful, non-judgmental stance:

> **John** was diagnosed with SAD three years ago. Even as an adolescent John noticed that his energy and motivation plummeted in the winter. He finds the season particularly bad this year. He uses light therapy but wants to understand and explore other ways to overcome SAD.
>
> John's therapist works with him on decreasing judgmental thinking. She explains how critical, judgmental thinking increases his depression and stirs up bad feelings. She encourages him to complete an exercise to see if his feelings about winter can be softened by *non-judgmental observation* in place of his habitual thinking style.

The exercise below highlights the difference between judgmental and non-judgmental thinking. John's example helps you to see how to start observing as an alternative to judging.

1. **Think about something that you've been evaluating negatively.**

2. **Write down each and every critical thought (see Table 18-1 for an example).**

3. **Notice how you feel when you're finished and write those feelings down (see Table 18-1 for an example).**

4. **Think about what you just wrote.**

5. **Now connect with your senses and describe the same information from Steps 2 and 3 as objectively as you can.**

   Write these experiences as they come to you. Don't worry about sentence structure, punctuation, or grammar. Check out Table 18-2 for an example of this step.

6. **Notice how you feel now and jot these feelings down (check out Table 18-2 for an example).**

Table 18-1	John's Critical State of Mind Form

Critical Thoughts

I hate winter. It's always bitter cold. I'm always insufferably cold. I hate leaving the house. Even just getting into my car, I'm freezing. At home, I turn the heat up so that I'm warmer, but then I get the darn gas bill and feel horrible. Most days are dreary, cloudy, and gray. The sun rises too late and sets too early. I hate the way the snow turns gray and dirty on the sides of the road. Winter seems to go on forever here. In the winter I can barely function. I'm constantly miserable, tired, and eat too much. I hate winter. Winter is utterly intolerable.

Feelings after Writing Critical Thoughts

I feel like I always do in the winter. Lousy. I must be crazy to continue living in this cold place. If I was a kid, I could just cry. But my mood is so low when I think about winter that I can hardly stand it.

Table 18-2	Observing State of Mind Form

Observations, Sensations, and Experiences

The temperature is cold. Today's sky has a variety of clouds of different shapes and sizes. A little sun occasionally pokes through between some of the clouds. When the wind blows and the temperature is low, I can feel my face get cold. The sensations of cold on my face are interesting. My face stings a bit, and I experience some numbness. When I go back into the house, I can feel the warmth. I see the sun beginning to set on the horizon. The clouds turn red and blue in the light. Off in the distance I can see the lights turning on in other homes and businesses.

Feelings after Writing Observations and Experiences

After describing without judging, I don't feel as bent out of shape about winter. My mood is pretty neutral really, but that's a whole lot better than feeling distraught, angry, and down. I noticed interesting sights like the lights at the end of the day. I rarely notice the beautiful parts of winter when I am so busy judging, and even the cold doesn't seem so horrible when I merely notice and describe the sensations. It's even a little interesting.

The examples in Tables 18-1 and 18-2 illustrate how judging and evaluating our experiences can contribute to a darkening mood. You can find blank copies of both the Critical State of Mind Form and the Observing State of Mind Form in Appendix A. Make some copies and fill them out on various issues that you find your mind judging, criticizing, and evaluating.

Even when you judge things overly positively, you can set up critical evaluations. For example, when you give excessive praise to kids for getting all As on their report cards, you can lead them to feeling more upset if they bring home a B or two. Or making too much about your recent successes at weight loss can set you up to experience self-disgust if you gain a few pounds.

Taking Thoughts Less Seriously

The depressed mind produces thoughts like a computer spitting out random numbers, codes, words, or whatever. The thoughts don't have to make sense, and they generally aren't even grounded in reality. But thoughts are just thoughts. They're not facts, and they don't represent so-called reality. We're not saying that your thoughts are crazy, but we're saying that when you listen to your thoughts and believe that they're real, you can easily fall into a trap.

Take a look at some of these thoughts that our clients, friends, colleagues, and even we've had from time to time. Try to imagine how you'd feel if you viewed these thoughts as facts:

- ✔ Winter is insufferable.

- ✔ I can already tell that this day will be miserable.

- ✔ There's no way I can succeed at this task.

- ✔ If I touch a doorknob, I know I'll get sick if I don't wash my hands right away.

- ✔ Nothing turns out well for me.

Of course, one approach to thoughts like these is to figure out how to examine the evidence that either supports or refutes them (discussed in Chapters 9 and 10). And examining the evidence is probably the best way to start. But another strategy is to simply realize that the vast majority of negatively charged thoughts are nothing more than thoughts.

When you notice thoughts tinged with self-loathing, self-degradation, negativity, despair, or other unnecessary emotionality attached, try the following suggestions:

- ✔ Sit back, close your eyes, and imagine writing your thoughts on a leaf. Then toss the leaf into a stream and watch it float away.

- ✔ Sit back, close your eyes, and imagine writing your thoughts on a cloud that you watch drift across the sky.

- ✔ Repeatedly say to yourself, "Thoughts are just thoughts . . . thoughts are just thoughts . . . thoughts are just thoughts. (Do you think our editors would let us keep typing " . . . thoughts are just thoughts for the next five pages? Probably not. Sigh.")

This exercise takes a little practice. But as you practice, you're likely to start viewing and relating to your thoughts a little differently. They lose some of their emotional charge, and you slowly but surely start to disengage and let go of such thoughts.

Understanding Self-Esteem

People with SAD quite often report having low self-esteem, especially during an active episode. So you may assume that what you need is a high self-esteem. If you walked into any bookstore and looked for the section on self-esteem, you'd see quite a selection that includes such alluring titles as the following:

- ✔ *31 Days to High Self-Esteem*
- ✔ *Ten Days to Self-Esteem*
- ✔ *Achieving High Self-Esteem*
- ✔ *I Love Me!*
- ✔ *I Am a Star! My Building High Self-Esteem Book*

The message is so appealing and seductive — and wrong. Now please realize that we don't intend to skewer these books or their authors; in fact, some of these publications contain good advice. At the same time, the message that high self-esteem solves your problems is dangerously misleading.

The next section tells you what's wrong with investing too much energy into your ego and self-esteem and then you get a lesson on an alternative to high self-esteem called *self-acceptance*.

Presenting the balloon theory of self-esteem

Think of self-esteem as a balloon. A balloon that has lost all of its air is a useless blob of rubber. It lies flat on the ground and can't fly in the air or float on the water. When people are depressed or in an episode of SAD, their self-esteem is like that deflated balloon — flat and non-functional.

On the other hand, a balloon with too much air is vulnerable to popping. If you carry such a balloon around, you have to be very careful not to let it touch much of anything for fear of it bursting and again becoming a useless piece of rubber. People whose egos are like the super inflated balloon appear quite full of themselves. They also tend to overreact to criticism and threats.

The surprising downside of self-esteem

One of our favorite psychologists, Dr. Roy Baumeister, wrote an article some years ago that laid out virtually irrefutable evidence concerning the dark side of high self-esteem; more specifically, he showed that people with *very high,* inflated self-esteem were prone to violence when their self-esteem was threatened or challenged by others. Work before then by other psychologists as well as ourselves, has now demonstrated that *overly* positive self-esteem appears linked to a wide range of problems including the following:

- Eating disorders
- Gambling
- Excessive spending
- Aggression
- Risky behaviors of various sorts
- Poor school performance

You want self-esteem that's like a balloon with just the right amount of air in it. A semi-full balloon can soar and dart among the clouds or bounce around a room. Such a balloon doesn't easily burst. If you carried a semi-full balloon around, you wouldn't worry about all the tiny bumps and scrapes that could cause it to pop.

An ego that is resilient and functional, like the semi-full balloon, is called *self-acceptance.* If you have self-acceptance, you can be aware of both your positive and negative qualities without too much worry about either. Bumps in the road in the form of threats or criticism won't burst your bubble. In the section below, we give you a strategy for achieving self-acceptance and the serenity that accompanies it.

We don't advocate that you work on lowering your self-esteem! Throughout this book we reject acts of self-degradation, self-loathing, and self-downing in all its various forms. At the same time, it's important to realize that inflated self-esteem contains surprising, hidden dangers.

Appreciating your friends

You can figure out how to accept yourself, in good times and bad, but it does take some practice. After all, you may have been practicing self-downing for awhile, so accepting yourself won't happen overnight either. A great way to start appreciating yourself is by looking at your friends. As you do, reflect on each one's strong points and what you like and enjoy about the person.

After you've thought about your friends' finest qualities, spend some time pondering their imperfections, flaws, and quirks — not as a way of dragging your friends down, but in order to appreciate that you fully accept your buddies *in spite* of their human blemishes. Don't forget to spend some time marveling at how you manage to treasure your friend in spite of all those imperfections. Then try to apply the same appreciation to *yourself.*

The following example illustrates how to do this exercise:

> **Cassandra** is experiencing another episode of SAD. She has gained a few pounds and thinks of herself as a worthless pig. She dwells on each and every one of her personal shortcomings. Her therapist suggests that she carry out the "Appreciating Friends" exercise (see Table 18-3). He asks her to name one of her best friends. She chooses Manuela. He tells her to divide a piece of paper into two columns labeled "Valued Characteristics" and "Imperfections," followed by some space to reflect on how much she appreciates her friend and how much she's bothered (or not) by her friend's imperfections. Then he asks her to try and apply the same lesson to herself.

Table 18-3 is Cassandra's Appreciating Friends Exercise.

Table 18-3	Cassandra's Appreciating Friends Exercise: Manuela
Valued Characteristics	*Imperfections*
Sense of humor — she's so funny!	Sometimes she gets pretty irritable.
Compassion — she'll do anything for her friends.	When she gets angry with someone, she can hold a grudge.
Empathy — she understands me better than anyone else does.	She's a little overweight.
We enjoy many of the same things.	She can't seem to keep a good relationship with a guy.
I love talking with her; she always has something interesting to say.	Sometimes she talks too long on the phone.
She's a very good person; she's helped me grow.	

In Table 18-3, Cassandra comes to the conclusion that she adores Manuela. They struggle with different things, but she doesn't think badly of Manuela for it. Cassandra's friend has plenty of flaws, but they don't matter to her at all. There's no one in the world that she can think of more highly than her friend Manuela. Cassandra decides that it's time to stop beating up on herself so much.

Do what Cassandra did. Divide a piece of paper into two columns labeled "Valued Characteristics" and "Imperfections." Add some lines beneath your table for reflections. Consider running this exercise on several of your very best friends. See if this exercise helps you gain a little more self-acceptance.

Focusing On Meditating and Mindfulness

Guess what? The other sections of this chapter have each addressed an element of a general practice that is sometimes referred to as mindfulness. *Mindfulness* is an ancient practice that's enjoyed a resurgence in popularity and interest in the past decade or more. Mindfulness involves practicing giving up judgment, accepting what can't be changed, and connecting with the present.

If you suffer from SAD, you may be wondering why you need to study mindfulness. Substantial research shows mindfulness can help people feel better who suffer from depression, chronic pain, anxiety, and other ailments. Evidence also supports the value of mindfulness in helping people prevent relapse following successful treatment of their depression. Therefore, mindfulness can help you deal with SAD and/or prevent relapses.

The other sections of this chapter have dealt with the more active steps of mindfulness you can take to change your thoughts and outlook. This section focuses on a more passive step: meditation.

Meditating for better health

Literally billions of people throughout the world have practiced some form of mindfulness. Monks, priests, medicine men, shamans, yoga instructors, as well as ladies in pink leotards at the gym. *Meditation* is one type of mindfulness that's embraced by a wide variety of religions. (Although many religions involve meditation, please realize that mindfulness and meditation can be practiced without any religious significance.)

Meditation describes a mental state of attention and concentration. Meditation takes on many different forms such as concentrating on breathing, focusing on a candle, contemplating on a particular subject, counting, humming, or repeating mantras. Many types of meditation are done in a seated pose although some are done while standing or even walking. Typically, eyes are closed or partially closed during meditation.

Meditation can help you if you suffer from SAD. The benefits of meditation are well documented. Multiple research studies have found that meditation decreases anxiety, depression, chronic pain, and improves health. Meditation suppresses the discharge of the body chemical cortisol, which has been implicated as a culprit in heart disease, high blood pressure, and stroke. Meditation can help boost immune systems. Meditation does more than decrease disease, pain, and negative moods; people who regularly meditate also report feeling calmer and happier than they did prior to starting their practice.

Meditating — no equipment required

Ready to sign up? Meditation doesn't require expensive equipment. You don't need lessons to begin. However, you do need to set aside some time for meditation and commit to regular practice. A few minutes a day is a good start and that short amount of time can reduce stress and lead to a greater sense of well being.

Some meditation can be done sitting, standing, or walking. We recommend sitting for the following exercise and being still, which enhances your sense of calmness.

Get going on a breathing meditation with the following tips:

- ✔ **Find a quiet spot.** You don't need a special room for meditation. Find somewhere you won't be disturbed by other people. Meditation can be done inside or outside.

- ✔ **Turn off the world.** You really can't meditate and watch the news on TV. Turn off the television, unplug your phones, and put your cell in silent mode. Listen to quiet music (please, no rap or heavy metal).

- ✔ **Sit on a cushion.** Any cushion or chair will do. However, you can go online or to a sporting goods store and purchase mats and pillows for meditation. The square mats are called *zabutans.* A smaller pillow to make sitting more comfortable, called a *zafu,* can also be purchased. Some people choose to sit on a couch or chair instead of a mat.

- ✔ **Find your sitting position.** You can sit for meditation in various ways. The important point to remember is to find a posture that you can maintain during the practice. So, after you sit, no wiggling around! Many people have trouble with sitting for long periods of time. Yoga exercises (see Chapter 15) can help strengthen and stretch the body in preparation for meditation.

- ✔ **Close your eyes and start to notice your breathing.** When you begin your meditation practice, you may notice that your mind starts to chatter. Keep coming back to your breathing and let the thoughts float away.

✔ **Keep focusing on breathing.** Try to let go of tension. Relax your muscles. Scan your body for any tightness and relax. Thoughts may intrude; let them go. You may wish to count your breaths from 1 to 10, then again. You can also repeat words or sounds. Feel the air pass through your body and into your lungs. Slow, deep, breaths. Let go of all tension; soften your eyes; let your face relax.

✔ **Sit quietly.** At first, aim for 5 or 10 minutes of practice. As you progress, you can increase the time gradually.

✔ **Be patient and kind to yourself.** Meditation takes practice. Results don't come instantly but are obtained over time. Many people report immediate feelings of relaxation, but the health benefits and sense of well being take longer.

Consider taking a class on meditation or going to a meditation retreat. Instruction can be very helpful. Getting support in the early stages of developing meditation practice increases your chance of enjoying, mastering, and continuing this important life skill.

Occasionally meditation evokes disturbing thoughts and/or feelings. If that happens to you, stop meditating! You may try again, but do so under the guidance of mental health professional trained in meditative techniques.

Presenting . . . the present

Most people who report experiencing anxiety, dread, and fear, focus on the future — one filled with imagined dreadful events. They worry about finances, failures, rejection, their kids, deadlines, and traffic accidents. There's no end of worries that you can put on your list. And probably less than 5 percent of the things people worry about ever happen. Perhaps even more importantly, when bad things do happen, people usually cope far better than they think they would.

People who experience depression and guilt usually dwell endlessly on past regrets. They wallow in self-accusation for not having done this or that, missing out on past opportunities, failing to reach goals, and childhoods that were traumatic or just disappointing. They go back to these events again and again in their minds, without realizing the past is truly passed. Re-experiencing the bad times in thoughts and images keeps people stuck.

Few present moments are all that bad. When you find your thinking immersed in the past or becoming anxious about the future, try to focus on what's happening now. Notice your breathing, notice how your chair feels, feel your feet on the floor. Focus on all the sights, sounds, and sensations that you're connecting with right now. Stay in the present. You'll feel much better.

Chapter 19

Living Happily after SAD

In This Chapter

▶ Getting the scoop on happiness

▶ Building better relationships

▶ Finding control in your life

▶ Exploring beneficial aspirations

*W*hat happens after you're no longer battling recurring episodes of SAD? Can you build on this absence of depression and find real happiness? You can find true happiness, and not only can you find happiness, but also you can sustain it, which adds one more tool to your arsenal for keeping SAD away forever. This chapter defines happiness as we see it — a deep feeling of contentment and overall peace — and tells you how to achieve this seemingly elusive state, regardless of whether you've suffered from SAD for a few months or off and on for decades.

This chapter helps you the most if you read it when you're not bogged down with depressed feelings. Therefore, first work on defeating SAD through the ideas in other chapters in this book and/or with professional help. Then you're ready to move beyond SAD.

Defining and Refinding Happiness

You probably don't spend a lot of time pondering what happiness is; most folks just assume they know. Or, perhaps, because of SAD's impact on your life, you're not so sure anymore. That's okay.

Philosophers, social scientists, and spiritual leaders have debated the happiness subject for centuries, and they still haven't got it worked out. They probably never will. Book publishers have capitalized on the confusion by providing answers in the form of dozens of books offering to give you the latest answer on how to live happily ever after.

We haven't written that book . . . yet. And we don't claim to have the final, definitive answer for what happiness is and how to get it. But we do have some pretty good ideas based on readings, research, and experience. Most opinions on what happiness is fall into one of two general areas:

✔ **Happiness is the pursuit of pleasure.** Some people define happiness as sensory pleasures, hedonistic pursuits, and indulgences. We call them the *Pleasure Pursuers*. For them, happiness is found in the first bite of a hot chocolate brownie topped with rich vanilla ice cream, smothered in fudge sauce. Hold on while we take a break. We'll be right back.

Okay, we're back now. The ice cream was great, but now we feel guilty about our splurge. The sensory delight was short-lived. That's one of many reasons that "happiness experts" often dismiss sensory pleasures as having little to do with "true happiness."

✔ **Happiness is the pursuit of meaning or purpose.** This camp is the *Meaning Makers* because they proclaim that true happiness can only be found by leading a meaningful, altruistic life filled with good works, higher values, and positive relationships. For them, happiness emerges from close, positive relationships, feeling grateful for life, participating in engaging work, exercising self-control, and contributing to humankind. The most extreme of the Meaning Makers suggest that your life's true purpose, meaning, and happiness can't be ascertained until after you die. Hmm.

Finding balance

In our humble opinion, at the extreme, both camps from the preceding sections are wrong. There's nothing wrong with seeking momentary pleasures as long as you're careful not to hurt anyone in the process. In fact, such pleasures are so important that we devote an entire chapter to them (see Chapter 16). At the same time, a life without meaning is well, meaningless. Relationships, values, and purpose form the foundation of a good life. People report greater happiness when they engage in helping others, bettering the world, and creating connections.

We believe happiness is an intricate balance of momentary sensory pleasures intertwined with a quest for meaning. So treat yourself with regular doses of self-indulgence whether it's ice cream, reading great novels, or getting a massage. At the same time, it's a pretty good idea to take stock of your life, evaluate your priorities, and make sure that you feel you have some purpose and meaning to your life's mission.

Now that you have a clearer idea of what happiness is, you may be wondering why you should bother taking steps toward happiness. Happiness is an anti-SAD elixir. It's pretty difficult to feel happy and profoundly sad at the same

Happy nuns live longer

Research on an often-cited study of nuns demonstrates that happiness likely leads to longevity. Why study nuns? Well, the great thing about studying nuns is that most aspects of their lives are pretty much the same — diet, stress, sleep patterns, spirituality, lifestyle, and so on. That fact makes it easier to study the effects of other specific variables like happiness.

More than 600 nuns born before 1917 were asked to participate in a large study on aging. Lucky for researchers from the University of Kentucky, 180 of these nuns had also written short autobiographies on taking their final vows in the 1930s (most were in their young 20s at the time). Their autobiographies were analyzed for how much positive content (signs of happiness) they contained. Autobiographies were also scrutinized for negative content. More than six decades later, nuns

who'd written the most positive content in their autobiographies were more likely to be alive. In fact, those women with the most positive content lived about *ten years* longer than nuns with the most negative content.

Does this study mean that happiness caused nuns to live much longer? Not necessarily, because it's always possible something else was responsible for this connection. However, we can say that these findings are strongly suggestive of the benefits of happiness, and alternative explanations for the results don't readily come to mind. If the link between happiness and longevity holds up, research will be needed to determine why it has that effect. Possibilities could include that happy people exercise more, eat healthier, and so on.

time. Finding ongoing pleasure and meaning in life can carry you through the darkest winter months! Researchers are constantly discovering new benefits of happiness. For example, numerous studies indicate that in general, happy people live longer (see the nearby sidebar, "Happy nuns live longer").

The health benefits of happiness

If happiness increases your lifespan, you may just think that happiness also can make you healthier. Certainly the reverse appears to be true — depression and anxiety have been strongly linked with various indicators of poor health, such as high blood pressure and heart disease. Preliminary studies have suggested that happiness and positive feelings are linked with fewer strokes, fewer injuries, lower blood pressure, and even more successful in vitro fertilization. One study looked at positive emotional style and the frequency of coming down with colds. People who reported greater happiness had fewer colds.

Furthermore, happy people are more able to handle the everyday hassles that everyone faces such as getting sick, paying bills, and dealing with losses. People who feel positive tend to have more ideas and flexible thinking. Flat out: Happiness is good for you!

Although we're sure that pharmaceutical companies are working feverishly to create happiness from a pill, no such drug exists at this time. Even if it did, somehow we think you're a lot better off if you pursue happiness through methods that we discuss in this chapter. In case you're wondering, antidepressant medications don't create happiness; they only alleviate depression.

Reclaiming Relationships

Relationships and social support contribute to people's sense of well being and happiness. Furthermore, connecting with people appears to improve health, extend life, and buffer against the effects of stress. Such relationships include intimate partnerships, close friends, memberships in organizations, coworkers, colleagues, and casual acquaintances. The more connections you have and the better the quality of those relationships, the better off you are.

When you were in the throes of SAD you may have withdrawn from people around you. When you don't feel good, the natural instinct is to pull the covers over your head and hibernate. You don't have the energy to venture forth and connect. This pullback can hurt your connections with friends and intimate partners alike.

Usually, when people get SAD, their partners feel empathetic — at first anyway. Most partners respond with caring behaviors and a lot of patience. But SAD can wear down even the most patient partner. A partner can feel hurt by your detachment and eventually respond by distancing from you as well.

And as understanding as your friends may try to be, after a while, they're likely to take your withdrawal personally and feel rejected. Then when your friends withdraw, you feel rejected too. That's how SAD does its work.

Relationship difficulties are common for people with or without SAD. You may have no symptoms of SAD whatsoever yet experience troubles communicating with your partner or friend. This section intends to help you connect more positively with your loved ones even if you've fully recovered from your SAD. Better connections help prevent new episodes.

Detecting difficulties in your relationships

Not everyone with a case of SAD experiences relationship turmoil. Some people get lucky, and their relationships glide along smoothly. However, sometimes storms brew underneath, and if you're not vigilant, you can start meeting some resistance in your relationships.

In this section, we tell you how to predict turmoil in your relationships and then quell the turbulence in your relationships *before* it's too late.

In the story that follows, you see how even after recovering from SAD, symptoms can reoccur and threaten a relationship in the process. Addressing the relationship issues can improve the relationship as well as provide an important strategy for preventing a new full-blown episode of SAD.

> **Carolyn** and **Richard** have been married for almost 30 years. They're finally retiring from their busy teaching jobs and looking forward to travel, spending more time with grandchildren, and pursuing their hobbies. Richard has suffered from recurring bouts of SAD over the years, and Carolyn hopes that having more leisure time decreases the stress he's been under and improves his mood.
>
> Now it's the first fall in 30 years that the buzz of the alarm clock does not yank them out of bed. Richard feels like staying warm for a while and hits the snooze button. Carolyn leaves him in bed — she's wide awake. She has plans to meet with her book club at the library and gets ready to go. When she returns, she's surprised to see Richard still in bed. She asks him if he's alright, and he gets irritated that she's bothering him. She leaves the room and worries that retirement may not be what she hoped for. Richard slumps into the living room and asks what's for breakfast. Carolyn, out of patience, snaps back.
>
> Richard recognizes that he's having a few early signs of SAD. He decides to go back to a therapist he'd seen with some success in the past. His therapist suggests that he fill out a SAD Relationship Analysis Exercise to see if there is a developing problem in his marriage.

Check out Table 19-1 for an example of Richard's exercise.

Table 19-1	Richard's SAD Relationship Analysis Exercise
Question	*Response*
Have I been more distant in my relationship lately, and, if so, does my partner (or friend) seem affected by that?	Honestly, I guess I've withdrawn and pulled back. I don't think I've been talking much with Carolyn either. When she brings something up, I've just been sitting there like a bump on a log and not contributing to the conversation. No wonder she's seemed a little distant lately.
Have I been less affectionate and warm lately? If I have, in what ways?	I have to admit that I haven't shown Carolyn much warmth or affection. I've just been focusing on my own misery. That must feel bad to her. I certainly haven't held her hand, touched her as much, or even given her hugs like I usually do in the spring and summer.

(continued)

Table 19-1 *(continued)*

Question	Response
Have I been cross, irritable, or critical with my partner (or friend)? If so, what have I been doing?	If I'm honest with myself, I guess I've been a bear. I've been jumpy, and snappy with Carolyn. She must be thinking she can't do anything right. If she messes up the smallest thing, I criticize it. I know it's because I've been feeling so miserable, but that's not a great reason to take it out on her.
Have I been doing fewer of the "nice" things that I usually do when I'm feeling better? Have I been complimenting my partner (or friend) less than usual; have I felt like I didn't have the energy to do favors? Are there positive actions that I just haven't been doing lately?	In all honesty, I don't think I've done much for my wife lately. I used to compliment her all the time, and I don't think I've done that in a month now. I used to routinely clean up after dinner even if I was the one to cook, and now I sit around like a slug after we're finished. I haven't even been pitching in on housework; instead I sit around and moan and groan. I haven't felt great, but I've been taking all that out on her.

Completing the SAD Relationship Analysis Exercise helped Richard see how his early symptoms of SAD were already starting to negatively impact Carolyn. He vowed to do something about his behavior while also getting some preemptive help for his SAD before it got serious. He tried some of the strategies in the next two sections.

If you have any concerns about your current relationship, take out a sheet of paper and write down the questions from Table 19-1. Spend some time thinking about them and write out your answers. Ask yourself if there are productive things (as shown in the following sections) you can do to overcome the problems you identified in your SAD Relationship Analysis Exercise.

Making communication effective

The act of talking to your partner or close friends about your life, your day, or your feelings, by itself is likely to improve your mood. But SAD can interfere with your desire to communicate. People who're depressed tend to have difficulty communicating. They commonly display the following behaviors:

✔ **Easily distracted:** SAD can make it harder for you to concentrate on a conversation. Some people with SAD say that they lose track of what a person is saying in the middle of a sentence.

✔ **Exaggerate the negative:** When you're down, you're likely to make mountains out of molehills. When your partner tells you she forgot to pay a bill, you immediately think of what this mistake will do to your credit rating, and that you'll likely be unable to buy that new car you want. This thought too easily triggers a flash of anger on your part.

✔ **Supersensitive to criticism:** SAD involves depression. When you're depressed, you look for information that confirms your low feelings. For example, if you get a compliment from someone, you wonder if that person wants something from you or is somehow trying to fool you. When there's a bit of feedback such as "Gee, you look tired today," the person with SAD may think, "I must look horrible, why is that person so mean?"

If any of the above problems pertain to you and your partner (whether you experience symptoms of SAD or not), start a regular routine called The Daily News. *The Daily News* is a strategy for improving the quality of the communication in your relationship. It's a set time that you and your partner can use for sharing the events of your day. By using certain rules, you can improve your listening skills and enhance the intimacy you feel toward each other.

Here's how it works:

1. **Make a regular time for The Daily News.**

   Write the time on your calendar. Be sure it's a convenient time and that you won't be interrupted. If something does come up, try to do The Daily News anyway or at worst, only put it off a little while. Make it a priority.

2. **Pick one person to start the conversation.**

   There's no prescribed topic here, but focus on the interesting events from your day instead of an emotionally charged conflict you've been having. For example, you may talk about a new work project, the traffic, or something you've read. Ideally, alternate who goes first. Let your partner talk for about 10 to 20 minutes. Decide ahead of time how long it will be. Try not to exceed the time limit.

3. **Listen.**

   To really listen, can be tough for a lot of people. You can listen better if the listener refrains from jumping off on a new topic. You can also listen better by showing empathy, nodding, repeating a few words to check if you got the message correctly, and summarizing what you heard. This part actually sounds easy, but it takes practice.

4. **Stay away from advice giving!**

   If your partner specifically asks for advice, you can consider giving a little. However, if you jump in unasked, it's easy to disrupt the flow and your partner can easily feel dismissed. The best way to give advice is actually by asking your partner for ideas that he or she may have for solving the problem. In other words, avoid thinking you have all the answers!

5. Avoid conflict.

The Daily News isn't the time to talk about complaints and what's wrong with each other. Don't allow The Daily News to ignite a fire between the two of you.

The Daily News can enhance your relationship if you practice it often. You can feel closer to your partner and warm feelings are likely to emerge. Good communication about everyday life prepares you to tackle more difficult topics when you need to. Let The Daily News become a regular habit before you try to deal with other, more problematic issues.

The Daily News strategy can also be used to strengthen friendships. Pam and Debbie used The Daily News to good advantage when they felt that their long-standing friendship was growing more distant.

> **Pam** and **Debbie** are stressed, busy professional women. They've been very close friends for the past 15 years. Debbie was grateful to Pam for suggesting light therapy for her SAD. However, in the past couple of years, Debbie and Pam had fallen into a habit of not connecting very often, especially so during the winter months. They realized that their friendship was strained and in jeopardy. To solve the problem, they changed "Daily" to "Weekly News" and started meeting on Saturday mornings for coffee. They used the same strategies as in the more frequent "Daily News" and found that their friendship quickly regained the feeling of closeness they both treasured.

Demonstrating true caring

If you have a friend, spouse, or partner, you probably care about that person. Perhaps you care a great deal. But the real question is how do you demonstrate your caring?

People often say that over time, "we just drifted apart." All too often, the drift starts by a gradual process of forgetting — in other words, forgetting to engage in positive exchanges with each other. Couples forget to give compliments, do nice things for each other, and plan enjoyable times together. It's much easier to notice things that people *do* than the things they *aren't* doing, so it's easy to drift apart without awareness that the process is happening until it's too late.

Ah, but once again, we have a solution for you! And it's a technique that almost sounds too simple to do any good. Frankly, when we first heard about it, we were "underwhelmed" with excitement about its potential to help relationships. We were dead wrong in our initial appraisal of the strategy — couples we've seen and thousands of couples who've tried it at the suggestion of their relationship therapists have found that this approach increases closeness and rekindles romance. So what is it? The originator of the technique (Dr. Richard Stuart) calls it *Caring Days*.

What's Caring Days? It's a technique in which you regularly insert small acts of caring into your relationship. These caring acts provide glue for your connections. Gary and Janet benefit from Caring Days:

> **Gary** and **Janet** recently celebrated their 25th wedding anniversary. Janet suffered from SAD off and on over the years. However, she sought therapy and has been free of all symptoms for the past four winters in a row. In general, she says her life is good. She and Gary have great jobs, they look forward to retirement in a few years, and their three adult children are all flourishing. Just one problem — Janet senses that she and Gary have been drifting apart for the past couple of years. They don't spend as much time together as they used to; they don't talk as much; and they feel more distant from each other.
>
> Janet remembers seeing the Caring Days exercise in *Seasonal Affective Disorder For Dummies* and asks Gary to do it with her.

Here's how Caring Days works:

1. **Have a discussion with your partner and brainstorm a list of specific actions or behaviors that may feel like caring or affection.**

   Even if just one of you feels that the behavior would indicate caring, jot it down. Here are a few guidelines for this list of caring behaviors:

   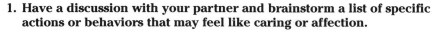

   - Each one needs to be very *clearly worded* and *specific* so that you know for sure if it has occurred. For example, instead of listing *be nice to me,* state that you'd feel cared about if your partner *ran an errand without being asked.*

   - Each action should be stated in positive terms, not negative. You may suggest *giving compliments* instead of *don't criticize me.*

   - Don't jot something down that you've fought about recently. Don't include a request for your partner to spend a few minutes talking on the phone with your mother when she calls if you've just had a blow up about it.

   - These behaviors should consist of fairly small, easy to carry out actions, not something huge and burdensome. An item of *leaving an endearing note* would be a lot better than *cleaning out the entire garage* that's been unattended to for the past nine years.

   - Ideally, the actions should be easily repeatable over and over again. For example, you can give many compliments, back rubs, and small gifts. The same wouldn't be true of getting a new puppy. Do that too many times and well . . .

2. **Get a sheet of paper and divide it into two columns.**

   In the left hand column, write down each of your "Caring Behaviors." List the name of the person who intends to carry it out as well. That means that each of you may have an identical item in your name, such as *give a backrub*.

3. **As each day comes to a close, jot down the date by every item that you noticed your partner having carried it out for you.**

   Your partner should do the same thing. If someone doesn't notice a particular item that was carried out, the partner can *ever so gently* point it out, and the date should then be noted. For example, you could say, "I guess you didn't notice that I took the car in for an oil change. It's no big deal; sometimes I don't notice things you do either."

4. **Pledge to do at least two of these behaviors every single day.**

   And it's desirable to aim for as many as four or five. You need not carry out each and every item, but do try to do a variety of them over time — don't just mindlessly repeat the same ones day after day.

Tape the Caring Days exercise somewhere that you won't fail to notice it. Sometimes that's on a bathroom mirror; some people prefer the refrigerator. Check out Table 19-2 for an example chart of Caring Days.

Table 19-2	Gary and Janet's Caring Days
Caring Behaviors	*Dates Carried Out*
Gary brings Janet flowers.	1-12; 2-6
Janet puts gas in Gary's car.	1-8; 1-23; 1-30
Gary puts gas in Janet's car.	1-12; 1-22; 2-5
Gary cooks a romantic meal.	1-30
Janet sends an endearing note or card.	1-22; 1-30; 2-6
Gary sends an endearing note or card.	2-4; 2-8
Gary rubs Janet's back.	1-30; 2-7
Janet rubs Gary's back.	1-30; 2-7
Gary calls Janet at work just to say he loves her.	1-23; 1-27; 2-4; 2-7
Gary plans a romantic date.	2-7
Janet prepares Gary breakfast in bed.	1-31; 2-8
Janet clears the snow from the front walk.	1-15, 2-1

After Gary and Janet have tried Caring Days for a few weeks, they notice that they feel closer to each other. They feel a new spark of romance as well. That's because they regularly feel cared about.

Our sample Caring Days exercise gives you some ideas for various caring behaviors. Continually add to your list until each of you has at least 15 items. The more, the better.

Regaining Control

SAD saps your sense of self-control. The SAD can seem to be controlling you. However, you can increase the sense of control over your life. As you do, your moods are less vulnerable to almost anything that happens to you from congested traffic to less light in the winter. See Chapters 7, 14, and 15 for more information about increasing the amount of control you feel.

Most people want to exercise some level of control. You can exert two types of control:

- ✔ **Internal control:** Self-control is like a muscle — the more you exercise it, the stronger it gets. Try eating one less French fry, get up without hitting the snooze button, save a little each paycheck no matter what, or postpone that trip to Vegas until you've paid off your credit cards. Be conscious of the act of self-control and pat yourself on the back each time you exercise it.

   Self-control also helps people do better. Folks who have a sense of self-control and the ability to delay gratification make more money, do better in academics, have more friends, and report greater levels of happiness.

- ✔ **External control:** Exert control over your life. Take part in the election process, (voting) — many elections have shown that each voter makes a difference. Also, consider keeping a daily calendar with daily and weekly goals and accomplishments. Many people forget what they've done on most days, whereas if you keep track, you may surprise yourself. Take control over your health by asking your doctor questions, reading up on any concerns, and doing your part to stay healthy through exercise and diet.

Having a sense of both types of control has proven to benefit both physical and emotional well-being. Numerous research studies support this notion. Therapy clients who believe that they're helpless and unable to change don't get better as quickly as people who believe they're capable of changing. Workers perform better if they believe that they have some voice in how to do their job. Post-surgical hospital patients use less pain medication when they have some degree of choice about how much and how often to administer the medication. Nursing home residents who were offered some control about when to eat and watch movies lived longer than others without these seemingly minor choices. Even cancer patients have worse outcomes if they feel helpless and without choices in the management of their disease.

Aging and control

For many older people, one of the most painful aspects of getting old is losing a sense of control over their lives. When old and sick, people often have to give up driving a car, traveling, shopping, or visiting with others. When people lose control, they feel helpless and depressed. This feeling is particularly strong when older people live in a nursing home. A study done in the '70s devised a clever way to look at how control affects the health of an elderly population.

Researchers studied three groups of residents in a nursing home. The first group was told that it could choose the frequency and length of time that a college student would stop by to visit. Researchers told a second group that it would have a college-aged visitor but wasn't given choices concerning how long or when the visit would occur. A third group had visitors pop in on a random schedule. A fourth group didn't get visits from the college students. When the study ended, the first group, that had control over the visitation times, was healthier and happier than the other groups.

Taking the "Me" out of Meaning

Psychologists have found that the more you focus on *yourself* (what shrinks call self-absorption), the more miserable you are. They've found that the more you worry about how you look, how you're doing, and what others are thinking about you, the more likely you are to feel depressed, anxious, and unhappy. And the more depressed and anxious you are, the more likely you are to spend time thinking about yourself. It's a vicious cycle.

The word *ruminate* captures this process rather nicely. People have a disturbing tendency to repeatedly chew over their worries, regrets, and sorrows. Again, it's a vicious cycle with misery as the outcome. But you can stop the cycle. Stopping the cycle is a little illogical — the less you focus on yourself, the happier that self becomes. In other words, taking the *me* out of *meaning* actually enhances your sense of purpose in life. The following sections help you focus on a path of meaning to take care of yourself.

Being grateful

Thank you for is such a common phrase, yet, these three words can have a powerful effect on your mood. If you're like most people, you may say thank you dozens of times at day. You probably use those words automatically, like saying "Hello, how are you?" and not waiting for an answer.

Gratitude is more than an automatic phrase like *thank you*. True gratitude allows you to more fully appreciate the good things in your life. Gratitude involves reflection and savoring of good fortune.

Studies have shown that consciously recording things that you feel grateful for increases positive feelings in more ways than you may guess. In one study, researchers asked various groups of people to keep a diary of what made them feel grateful. These folks reported improved sleep, fewer health complaints, better connections with people, more optimism, and increased feelings of well being.

Start making a habit out of recording what you feel grateful for. Use a small pocket-sized notebook. Reflect a few moments on each new item. These events don't need to be grand; everyday occurrences like a flower in the springtime, a hug from a friend, or a great, unexpected parking place are just fine. Just jot down whatever positive experiences you have — large or small. From time to time review your list. You don't even have to perform this exercise every day. Even once a week can bring you benefits.

Finding the kind in humankind

Helping others can help you take the focus off yourself. Most people report an increased sense of satisfaction and well being when they do nice things for someone else. Through the smallest of actions to larger ones, it's a good idea to make the world a little better place.

People who are charitable tend to be well liked by others. They feel a stronger sense of interconnection and fellowship with humankind. Often charitable acts are performed with people who have less than you. Thus, such acts lead to greater appreciation of your own life and yes, gratitude. So the circle of gratitude and kindness stops the cycle of self-focus, rumination, and emotional distress.

You may wonder how you can get started. Good question. Here's just a partial list:

- ✔ Check the Red Cross Web site at www.redcross.org/donate/volunteer. You can even volunteer online. It can direct you to local as well as worldwide efforts.

- ✔ Volunteer at your local Humane Society. (Our dogs like that one.)

- ✔ Check out www.volunteermatch.org. It has a long list of needs for volunteers in a wide range of areas.

- ✔ Check with a local senior center and volunteer to teach a class or deliver meals to shut-ins.

 ✔ Become a Big Brother or Big Sister.

 ✔ Pick up litter in your neighborhood; better yet, organize a litter group in your area.

 ✔ Volunteer to tutor at a school or with an adult who wants to learn to read (www.literacy.org).

 ✔ Donate blood.

 ✔ Write a heartfelt thank-you note to someone.

 ✔ Check out www.actsofkindness.org.

 ✔ Help out a neighbor.

No doubt, you lead a busy life. You may think that you don't have time for such acts of kindness. But helping someone with his groceries or picking up a little neighborhood trash doesn't take much time. You may find yourself more satisfied and happier if you infuse a little more kindness into your life.

Part VI
The Part of Tens

The 5th Wave   By Rich Tennant

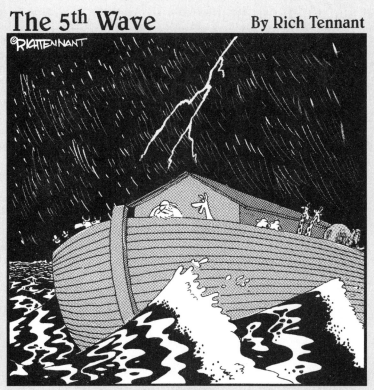

"Hey, look on the bright side. The sun will come out again in only 40 days or so."

In this part . . .

Take a look at the chapters in this part for quick advice and ideas that you can implement right away to help battle your seasonal affective disorder (SAD). We start by telling you ten ways for bringing more light into your life. And then you get some tips on dealing with bad moods. The last two chapters of this part guide you in helping someone you love — child or adult — with SAD.

Chapter 20

Ten Ways to Get More Light

*P*eople with seasonal affective disorder (SAD) usually profit from increased exposure to light. Of course shopping for a bright light box is one way to add more light to your life (see Chapter 5 for complete details about light therapy). After light therapy, SAD sufferers typically report improved mood, more energy, and fewer food cravings.

In this chapter, you get quick ways for increasing your exposure to light in other ways. You may find that these strategies suffice, although they're more likely to merely lessen the amount of time you need light therapy each day.

Greeting the Day

Before showering or eating breakfast, greet the day and the sun. Stand in front of a window; open the curtains, and face the outdoors. Even if your window faces the side of an old, deteriorating brick office building, look toward the sky. Slowly fill your lungs with air and hold the breath for a few moments. Then ever so slowly let the air release. Repeat this breath four or five times.

Going Outside

News flash. The sun is outside. Because the sun is the brightest source of light around, take every opportunity to bask in it — yes, even during the winter. And, of course, don't forget sunscreen.

Here are a few ways to work in some extra sun each day:

- ✔ Walk somewhere on your lunch break. You get the double bonus of extra exercise.
- ✔ Park a short walk from wherever you're headed so you spend an extra minute or two outside.
- ✔ Take a brief walk in the early afternoon. Outside breaks can provide a significant boost in your exposure to light.

Even on the coldest of days, you can get yourself outside for a few minutes several times a day.

You can get almost ten times as much light on a cloudy day as you do in a typical inside office. On a sunny day, your light exposure outside can reach as much as 25 times more than an inside space.

Finding an Outdoor Sport

People who engage in winter sports generally like winter. But if you have SAD, you probably don't like winter so much. Nonetheless, just try finding a winter sport that fits your fancy. Possibilities include ice skating, skiing, hiking, and snowboarding.

For the athletically challenged, snow shoeing is a good option. It's a lot harder to fall on huge snowshoes than skis. The exercise of picking your feet up and tromping through the snow keeps you warm. And exercise itself is very helpful for any type of depression, including SAD. See Chapter 15 for more information on the benefits of exercise.

Planting a Garden

Many people with really serious cases of SAD live in places where it may not be realistic to plant a garden in the winter. Most plants don't do well in freezing weather. And it really helps if the ground isn't frozen solid when you want to plant.

However, you can grow various house plants in pots inside. How does that get you more light? Well, you put your plants near windows and tend to them often.

Try planting an herb or two that you like to use in your cooking. Consult with your local garden center for ideas.

Brightening Up Your Home

You can add brightness to your home in a host of ways. Consider light-colored paint on your walls that reflect more light back into the room. If you like darker colors, consider three walls painted light and one a deeper hue.

You can also add light fixtures. Yes, saving energy is a good idea, but when you have SAD, you're allowed to turn up the lights — at least when you're in the room!

Energy-saving light bulbs can give more light and still consume less electricity.

Brightening Up Your Workplace

If you have SAD and sit in one area most of the day, consider buying a small light box for your desk (see Chapter 5). Even though it may not put out a full, recommended 10,000 lux, you can benefit from longer exposures to lesser amounts of lux. In addition, if moving your workspace closer to a window is possible, try that suggestion. If not, get outside more often (see "Going Outside" earlier in this chapter). Take part of your breaks as brief excursions outside. A few deep breaths in the parking lot work wonders. But don't stand right next to the tailpipe of a bus while you're breathing!

Plan a Cozy Spot

SAD sufferers complain about feeling cold much of the time. If you suffer from coldness, too, try these suggestions:

1. **Find an area in your house where you can curl up under an afghan (hopefully knitted by your grandmother).**

2. **Have a bright light shining on the space.**

3. **Take a few minutes during the day to unwind.**

   Read a magazine article or a few pages of your favorite novel. You may even have some favorite poetry or scriptures you enjoy rereading. You can also space out, meditate, or take a power nap.

4. **Sit and rejuvenate.**

Looking through Windows

Conveniently enough, most houses and many offices have windows. People habitually walk right by these windows without bothering even to glance out of them. If you suffer from SAD, that's a mistake. Whether you have a great view of the mountains (okay, we admit that we do) or just a parking lot, make a new habit of looking out your windows. Stand close to the glass and gaze a while.

Keeping Track of Light

You may be able prevent the emergence of a full-blown case of SAD merely by increasing your exposure to natural light. However, it takes a sustained effort to do so.

Review the list of ideas in this chapter and make a plan to try several of them each and every day. Then monitor (or even keep a journal of) the effects of increased light on your moods, your energy, and your food cravings.

Traveling to the Sun

In the winter, the sunlight travels to another part of the globe. Okay, technically the globe is the actual object shifting position. But you can travel to where the sunlight is. Consider taking a winter vacation to somewhere sunny. If you're in the Northern Hemisphere, go south. If you live in the Southern Hemisphere, go north for the winter. A winter sun break may just give you enough lift to get through the dark days.

Chapter 21

Ten Quick Ways Out of a Bad Mood

. . . .

In This Chapter

▶ Realizing the difference between SAD and a bad mood

▶ Using physical strategies to increase your good moods

▶ Surrounding yourself with positive people, pets, and things

. . . .

Seasonal affective disorder (SAD) is more than a bad mood. SAD without treatment can last for weeks or months. By contrast, bad moods may last a few minutes, hours, or occasionally a day or more. Bad moods are like a storm blowing through; depression (including SAD) is like an entire winter season.

However, people prone to any type of depression experience bad moods just like everyone else. Bad moods can deepen an ongoing episode of SAD. Or, if you're not in the middle of SAD, bad moods are simply, well, bad. In this chapter, you look at some quick ways out of a bad mood.

Using Your Head

Some quick hit strategies involve cognitive therapy, and it can sometimes do the trick for a bad mood. (Chapters 9 and 10 discuss the use of cognitive therapy for the treatment of SAD.) Essentially these techniques involve answering a few questions when you find yourself in a bad mood:

✔ Am I upset about something that is likely to look less important in a few weeks (or even months)?

✔ Am I making too much out of something that's happened?

✔ Is there a better way for me to handle what's been upsetting me?

✔ How have I gotten through moods like this before?

✔ Does being in a bad mood help me get through what's happening?

Take your answers to these questions for helping you view what's been going on in a different way. You're likely to find yourself feeling a little more optimistic about your situation.

Try Breathing

Sometimes bad moods feel like running out of gas. Oxygen fuels the body, and fueling up sometimes snaps you into a better mood. If you need a positive burst of energy, here's a quick breathing technique:

1. **Stand up straight and tall.**

2. **Let your arms hang down at your sides and exhale completely.**

3. **Slowly raise your arms out to the side while keeping them straight.**

   Inhale until your hands meet high over your head.

4. **As your hands point toward the ceiling, tilt your head up slightly.**

   Hold your breath a moment.

5. **Slowly exhale as you lower your arms back down to your side.**

   Repeat this breathing exercise five times.

Pumping Your Heart

Bad moods slow down the body and the mind. But you can use exercise intermittently to deal with dark moods. The best exercises involve making your heart pump faster. You can accomplish this goal by a fast walk, jogging in place, or jumping rope. Darn near anything that speeds up your heart and circulation for 10 or 15 minutes should suffice.

Chapter 15 tells you more about exercise to counteract depression.

Reading to Distract the Mind

If you like to read, having a few well-written novels around may be able to bust you out of your mood. For us, nothing beats being immersed in a really good story — whether it involves mystery, humor, drama, or intrigue. It's very difficult to remain in a miserable state of mind when you let your imagination travel with a great author for a while.

Napping Away Moods

Sleeping too much is often a symptom of depression, especially SAD. At the same time, a five- or ten-minute power nap, sometimes gives you a kick start.

If you aren't sleeping excessively already, consider taking a short snooze when a bad mood creeps up on you. But again, be careful. Don't resort to napping frequently and excessively if you're experiencing a full-blown episode of SAD. Try the other suggestions in this chapter.

Connecting with Friends

When you're sad or feeling down, reach out and connect with others. You can confess that you're not feeling at the top of your game, but don't dwell on the negative. Try recalling or reminiscing about previous good times or ask your friends and family what's been going on with them. Humans are social, and studies show that when they connect with each other, they do better.

Entertaining New Moods

Your moods tell you to avoid enjoyable activities because bad moods make you think that nothing gives you pleasure. However, if you push yourself to go ahead with something that you usually enjoy, your moods are likely to improve.

Do something that you enjoy. Eat chocolate (but not too much!), dance, sing, see a new movie, go bowling, climb a mountain. See Chapter 16 for more ideas about pleasurable activities.

Playing with Pets

Petting animals has been proven to decrease blood pressure and improve your mood. If you're feeling sad, pet something fuzzy. Dogs, cats, gerbils, or guinea pigs will do. (Though some would disagree, we suspect that snakes, lizards, and spiders just won't work for most folks.) If you don't have a pet, you can visit the pet stores for a little petting time.

You may also consider getting a pet. Before you do, though, invite a pet-owning friend over for a visit with pet in tow. This step can help you see how owning a pet really works and if you're cut out for pet ownership. You could also consider volunteering at your local Humane Society. It always has a need for people willing to help.

If you volunteer at a Humane Society, you may end up taking one of the animals home with you! Actually, that's not a bad idea, if you're ready, because people with pets tend to live longer and feel happier.

Doing Good

When you feel down, your thoughts inevitably focus on your own troubles. Try looking outside of yourself. Find something that you can do to help others. It doesn't have to be a huge project. Just try these simple ideas:

- Send someone a thank-you card.
- Compliment a friend or coworker.
- Tell your partner how much you appreciate him or her.
- Give someone a hug.

When you extend yourself to others, your thoughts and moods shift — and so may theirs!

Using Acceptance to Ease Your Moods

Chapter 18 discusses the concepts of acceptance and mindfulness as ways to defeat SAD. You can use a brief version of these techniques to change your moods for the better. The next time you feel a bad mood coming on, try to

1. **Notice your breathing; feel the air going through your nostrils into your lungs and out again.**

2. **Notice the sensations in your body as if you were preparing a report for a science project.**

3. **Look around you and describe your environment — without judgment or criticism.**

4. **Return to noticing your breathing.**

5. **Study your moods and bodily sensations.**

   Realize that all bad moods pass; just give it a little time.

Chapter 22

Ten Ways to Help People with SAD

*I*f you don't suffer from seasonal affective disorder (SAD), winters may be a blast. Possibly you love skiing, skating, snow, sleet, and slush. But if someone you're close to has SAD, you may find yourself out of synch. In this chapter, you discover how to take care of someone with SAD by first understanding the disorder and then by knowing what to do to help. Armed with this information, you're more likely to understand and support your loved one.

Understanding SAD

Sometimes people either hide the symptoms they're experiencing, or their symptoms are quite mild and not easy to detect. Nevertheless, SAD disrupts and disturbs people's lives, and it's good to know what to look for. Pay attention to the following signs (especially if they increase in the fall and decrease in the spring):

- Complaining about feeling depressed, hopeless, or sad (especially with the onset of fall)
- Difficulty awakening in the morning
- Increased irritability
- Lowered motivation
- Problems concentrating
- Weight gain
- Withdrawal

Knowing about and understanding SAD are your first weapons in the arsenal you need to help your loved one break the cycle of SAD.

Listening to SAD

One of the most useful things you can do for someone who has any type of depression, including SAD is to listen. However, you may think that listening is a passive skill — people talk, and you hear them. But that's really not the case. People only truly feel heard when you listen actively.

To practice active listening, follow these steps:

1. **Pay close attention to what's being said.**

2. **Ask questions to help the person elaborate and clarify.**

3. **Express some concern and empathy.**

4. **Give your full attention and be sure to use nonverbals.**

   Nonverbal communication uses good eye contact, head nods (psychologists' favorite), and facial expressions. If you hear an especially poignant point, you may touch the person lightly on the shoulder or arm to show your concern.

Don't be working on your e-mail or watching television while the person is talking. Set aside some quality time to listen to your loved one with SAD.

Caring without Taking Care Of

The sections in this chapter are ways to show your loved ones that you care without doing everything for them. As the preceding section states, you want to listen to your loved one — that's one way of saying you care.

Actually solving the problem of SAD isn't up to you. People who have SAD ultimately must take responsibility for dealing with the problem. This book may be a very helpful start. Certainly consider giving a copy to the ones you care about if you think SAD is involved — but you can't do the reading for them!

Walking with SAD

Exercise really helps decrease the symptoms of SAD. You can encourage a loved one to exercise, but if you do, it's even better if you offer to do it together.

Here are a few fun suggestions:

- ✔ Join a gym and go together.
- ✔ Take a yoga or Pilates class.
- ✔ Do water aerobics.
- ✔ Take long walks together frequently — remember that increased sunlight, even on cloudy days, boosts the value of exercise further.

On really cold days, dress warmly and come back for a cup of hot tea or coffee (we'd say hot chocolate, but there's that weight gain problem . . .).

Helping Out

People with SAD often feel overwhelmed. Everyday tasks seem monumental. Sometimes helping out helps a little. Fortunately, with treatment, SAD usually improves within a few weeks so you probably won't have to keep your efforts up for too long.

No task is too small! For SAD sufferers, even the easiest task can seem huge. Doing a few small things for your loves ones may yield a big sense of relief for them. Simple tasks you can do include

- ✔ Going grocery shopping
- ✔ Cleaning their house or even just doing the dishes
- ✔ Running some extra errands (and taking them along)
- ✔ Balancing their checkbook
- ✔ Taking their car in for service
- ✔ Baby-sitting their kids
- ✔ Preparing a nice meal for them

Sometimes when people are SAD they don't remember to show appreciation. Continue your efforts in spite of that apparent snub and see the section "Knowing It's Not About You" later in this chapter.

Don't go overboard in helping someone with SAD. Although you can do some nice, helpful things, you don't want to take over all responsibilities. Doing too much could actually increase the person's sense of helplessness and dependency.

Recommending Help

If you're concerned about someone who has SAD, encourage the person to get help. Some people believe that emotional problems like SAD aren't treatable, but that's just not true. Many successful treatments are outlined in this book. If your loved one is willing to consider psychotherapy, you can help look for a qualified person (covered in Chapter 4). If lights look like the brightest option, you can help shop for lights with your friend (see Chapter 5 for more on light therapy).

Holding Criticism in Check

When people you care about are depressed, the circumstances can be pretty frustrating. Someone who previously appeared very competent may complain of feeling helpless. Another common symptom is irritability.

 Being around someone who's frequently irritable or who acts helpless when you know that isn't true isn't a lot of fun. In such cases, you may be tempted to find fault and criticize, but that won't help you or your loved one. Do your best to hold your tongue and recommend seeking help.

Providing Information

Maybe your loved one doesn't want to read an entire book like this one on SAD (hard to believe, but we're sure it's possible). You can ask the person to read a few relevant pages and sections. That's actually one of the great things about *For Dummies* books — you can read the chapters in any order you wish and still know what's going on.

You can also help the person with SAD find some resources on the Internet. Check out Appendix B for further resources. Information is out there, and tossing it someone's way won't hurt. (Oh, and the term *tossing,* meant gently handing it over, not flinging the book in someone's face.)

Knowing It's Not about You

People with SAD frequently get irritable. They don't act like themselves. Sometimes they withdraw and even reject the people that they truly care about. Do these responses mean they no longer care about you?

No! SAD is a mood disorder. People in chronically depressed moods don't think straight. They do things that they wouldn't normally do. So, try your best not to take their behaviors personally. Your loved ones' SAD really isn't about you. That doesn't mean you have to like the way they are acting; it just means you don't have to make yourself miserable too.

Not taking things personally doesn't mean you should put up with abuse. Ultimately the ones you care about need to do something to help themselves. In the meantime, cut them some slack unless their behavior gets outrageous. Fortunately, few people with SAD go to such extremes.

Taking Care of Yourself

Oh, let's not forget this last section. Do take care of yourself. Being a care-taker is hard work. Do what you can to be helpful for your loved one. Listen; try not to criticize or get angry; provide information; and take the tips in this chapter. Make sure that you don't let yourself fall into depression, too.

Stay connected with your friends. Exercise and eat right, take your vitamins. Get enough sleep. Make sure that you find ways to bring pleasure into your life. Realize that helping your loved one has limits. You can only do what you can do. If you find yourself struggling with difficult reactions, consider talking to a mental health professional to help you cope.

Chapter 23

Ten Ways to Help a Kid with SAD

In This Chapter

▶ Figuring out how to care for your child

▶ Keeping kids healthy with SAD strategies

▶ Considering the pros and cons of medication as a treatment option

*A*dults diagnosed with seasonal affective disorder (SAD) often report that they felt worse during the winter even as children. And studies have shown that children can and do experience full-blown SAD. In this chapter, we provide information about SAD symptoms in children and what to do if you see those symptoms in a child you care about.

Recognizing Kids with SAD

Recognizing that SAD exists in kids is one way to help. Children and adolescents with SAD suffer from many of the same symptoms as adults with SAD (see Chapter 2 for more info on symptoms). Typically, they lack energy, gain weight, appear moody, and show less motivation than usual. And of course these symptoms heighten during the winter months and subside during the onset of spring. Other common symptoms of SAD in kids can include

✔ Frequent tearfulness

✔ Social isolation

✔ A drop in grades

✔ Minor physical complaints like headaches and stomachaches

✔ Low self-esteem

✔ Overly sensitive to rejection

✔ Increased complaints about going to school

✔ Boredom

Wait! Don't these symptoms sound like almost every teenager on the planet? Well, it's true that adolescents tend to sleep more than other humans; they complain of boredom, they don't like rejection, and they're often a little on the rude side of things. But adolescents who don't have SAD function pretty well around their friends and show reasonable enthusiasm for fun and activities.

If your child is school age, then you may assume that SAD-like behavior is nothing more than a reaction to school getting into full swing in the fall. This scenario may be the case. However, if your child normally does well early and late in the school year (when the weather is nicer), but then has slipping grades as the days darken and the weather turns colder, SAD may be a factor.

SAD rarely appears in children below the age of 10 or so, and if it does, it can be difficult to recognize and distinguish from other types of problems. If you have concerns, take your child for an evaluation (see "Looking for Physical Problems" later in this chapter).

Getting Help for Yourself First

When you're sitting on the runway waiting for takeoff, the flight attendants give you safety instructions. These instructions include telling you to put your oxygen mask on first, before you assist a child sitting next to you. That's because without your own oxygen, you won't be able to help the kid.

The same principle is true for depression and SAD. If you suffer from any type of depression, including SAD, you need to get help for yourself first. Considerable research has shown that when parents or caregivers overcome their own depression, their kids do better. In fact, for some children who appear to be depressed, no treatment is necessary other than having their parents improve.

Looking for Physical Problems

If you have concerns about a child who suffers from a lack of energy, moodiness, and apathy, you need to check with your child's pediatrician or other healthcare provider. These symptoms can be an indication of a physical malady such as diabetes, allergies, or infections. In most cases, the doctor won't find any serious problems, but this possibility needs to be checked.

Checking Out Other Problems

After ruling out physical causes (see the preceding section), you still can't assume that a child has SAD. If you do rule out physical issues, then start looking for other problems that may be causing your child's behavior. Here are a few tips:

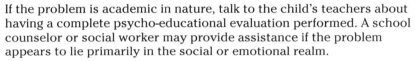

- ✔ **Talk with the child's teacher and school counselor.** Ask these folks how your kid is doing academically, socially, and emotionally. Are there any problems with paying attention, getting along with other kids, or learning?

- ✔ **Ask your child about any recent problems with friends or romantic relationships.** Breakups are difficult.

  If the problem is academic in nature, talk to the child's teachers about having a complete psycho-educational evaluation performed. A school counselor or social worker may provide assistance if the problem appears to lie primarily in the social or emotional realm.

Childhood disorders are quite varied and complex. Sometimes, they overlap with each other and/or occur in combination. Some childhood difficulties look like or can be confused with SAD. The list below contains those troubles that could mask as SAD. This list isn't complete and doesn't provide a comprehensive review of symptoms. We show it merely to illustrate the complexity of distinguishing SAD from other childhood maladies.

- ✔ **Attention Deficit Disorder:** This problem involves distractibility and inattentiveness. Children with SAD are also commonly inattentive.

- ✔ **Learning disabilities:** Children with learning disabilities seem bright, but don't always do as well as you'd expect in school. Children with SAD frequently underachieve.

- ✔ **Anxiety Disorder:** Kids with this type of emotional problem are usually nervous, anxious, and reluctant to attend school. Children with SAD often ask to stay home from school.

- ✔ **Autistic Spectrum Disorders (including Asperger's and Pervasive Developmental Disorder):** No one knows why for sure, but this diagnostic category is more common than in the past. Children with mild forms of this disorder may have trouble relating to other kids, responding well to discipline, and being overly sensitive to change. Children with SAD can demonstrate some of these same signs. Children with severe forms of this diagnosis are less likely to be confused with SAD.

The child's issue is likely to improve within a few months of intervention by the school. However, if you don't see progress, a more sophisticated diagnosis and intervention may be warranted. Consider seeking additional private help through a school or clinical psychologist.

Bullying Makes Kids Sad Too

Bullies don't cause SAD, but kids who are victims of bullies often become depressed. Some signs to look for include

✔ Not wanting to go to school

✔ Looking hopeless

✔ Complaining of fatigue

Because school starts in the fall, you may assume that your child has an emerging case of SAD. So, it's important to check with the child and the child's teachers to see if bullying is part of the picture. A good school counselor can probably help intervene if that's the case.

Your child may fear revealing this information, which is why you want to check with teachers and counselors. You may also consider going to the school to observe on a few days.

Shining Light on Kids with SAD

Perhaps you're wondering if light works as well for kids as it does for adults. Studies have shown that it does.

Pay especially close attention to your kids during therapy to make sure that they don't stare directly into the lights — that can damage their eyes. For more info on light therapy, check out Chapter 5.

An intriguing possibility for light therapy is a dawn simulator (see Chapter 5). Adolescents are notorious for their difficulty in awakening at a reasonable time in the morning (well, and some adults, too). Experts believe that adolescents in general may have more trouble regulating their biological clocks than adults. Dawn simulation just may help them reset their clocks to be in synch with the rest of the world.

Don't forget the great outdoors as a source of light for kids in the winter. Anything you can do to get them outside during the day is great.

Eating Better

Let's face it: Kids like junk food. SAD sufferers crave carbohydrates, and carbs are abundant in junk food. If you know a child with SAD, make sure to monitor food intake. Comb the kitchen and refrigerator and discard the tempting junk. Make sure you have healthy snacks available as alternatives.

Maintaining Healthy Sleeping Rituals

Most folks with SAD oversleep during the winter months. That can be a real problem for kids who have to get up and go to school. For better sleeping rituals try out these tips:

✔ Establish a regular bedtime routine.

✔ Make sure that pre-bedtime activities aren't too stimulating.

✔ Avoid eating dinner late because eating too much before bed can interfere with sleep.

✔ Provide a dawn simulator in your child's room (see Chapter 5).

✔ Have everything organized and ready to go the night before to minimize morning delays.

Incorporating Exercise

All children need exercise and especially folks with SAD. As with adults, a problem for kids with SAD is motivating them to get moving. Give children a choice of activities, but make sure they do something.

Choosing activities and sports that can be practiced on a lifelong basis is an especially smart move. Such sports include tennis, swimming, skating, skiing, dancing, and running. You get double bang for your buck if it's an outdoor sport that exposes the kid to a little sunlight.

Thinking about Medications

Some children need and benefit from medication. However, you may not want to try medications before trying a variety of other strategies first.

Various studies have shown that antidepressant medication with kids poses a small increased risk of suicide. Furthermore, people have concerns about the long-term effects of medication on a developing brain — these effects simply aren't known with certainty.

Primary alternatives to medications usually work just fine for kids. These options include

- ✔ Increased exercise
- ✔ Light therapy
- ✔ Individual psychotherapy (preferably cognitive-behavioral therapy — see Chapters 9 and 10). Therapists may recommend involving the whole family.

If you have concerns about a child who may have SAD, don't wait very long before seeking professional assistance. SAD and other emotional disorders in kids can be serious and warrant a consultation with a mental health professional.

Appendix A

SAD Forms for You

● ●

*I*n this appendix, you find several forms referenced throughout this book. Each includes a brief set of instructions and points you to the chapter where the form was first referenced in the book. You may photocopy these forms as needed, or use them as models to create your own personalized forms.

Food and Trigger Diary

In Chapter 7, we discuss the role of diet in SAD. The Food and Trigger Diary can help you analyze your eating patterns and spot trouble spots. After you've tracked your eating habits for a week or two, you can see what kind of events and moods trigger overeating, and you can develop a game plan for dealing with them. Here are the steps to creating your own diary:

1. **In the first column of this form, every time you eat or you're tempted to eat something, write down the day and time.**

2. **In column two, write down what was happening at the time from Column 1.**

   For example, if you crave food when you watch television or drive home from work, note what you were doing. If it's simply a meal time and nothing else was going on, just record *breakfast, lunch,* or *dinner.*

3. **Jot down your mood or what you were feeling in the third column.**

   See Chapter 9 for more information about feeling words.

4. **Record everything you ate and approximately what quantity (serving size or calories) in the last column.**

   If you craved food, but didn't eat it, write that down too.

5. **At the end of each day, under *My Reflections,* write a few sentences about your observations.**

   Try not to judge yourself too harshly, but record what you discovered from your diary.

Table A-1		Food and Trigger Diary	
Day/Time	*Event*	*Mood*	*Food or Craving*

My Reflections

Day/Time	*Event*	*Mood*	*Food or Craving*

My Reflections

Day/Time	*Event*	*Mood*	*Food or Craving*

My Reflections

Cost/Benefit Analysis

When you contemplate changing something or making a decision, you may experience some reluctance or ambivalence in committing to the change. A cost/benefit analysis helps you make the decision and motivates your efforts. You can use this exercise with a thought you're struggling with, your diet, or whatever you're thinking about changing. See Chapters 7 and 10 for examples of this approach. Here's the quick rundown:

1. **At the top of the form, write your goal, problematic thought, or decision that you're pondering.**

2. **In the left hand column, write about all the conceivable costs of making the changes you want to make.**

   Put down your deepest fears and concerns.

3. **In the right-hand column, write down all the imaginable benefits that your goal can bring you.**

   Don't be afraid to be creative.

4. **Under *My Reflections,* record what your cost/benefit analysis taught you.**

   In this section, include your thoughts about whether there's any way to minimize the costs.

Table A-2	Cost/Benefit Analysis
Goal, problematic thought, or decision:	
Costs	*Benefits*
My Reflections	

SAD Thought Tracker

A core part of cognitive therapy involves discovering the kinds of problematic thoughts you have and the events that trigger them, as well as the feelings and sensations you experience as a result of those thoughts. Use a SAD Thought Tracker to reveal the connections between your feelings, events, and thoughts when you experience distress. Please see Chapters 9 and 10 for more information about how SAD Thought Trackers can help you. Here's how a SAD Thought Tracker works:

1. **In the first column, *Feelings and Sensations*, write down both your body's sensations and a feeling word that describes those sensations.**

   Also rate the feeling words for intensity from 1 (very mild) to 100 (extremely intense or severe). You may have more than one feeling and/or sensations. Write them all here and rate the feeling.

2. **In the second column, *Events*, write down what you think may have triggered the feelings and sensations.**

   Ask yourself what was going on. Usually events involve something that happens to you. But sometimes, what gets everything rolling is a daydream or an image that floats into your mind.

3. **In the last column, *Thoughts or Interpretations*, record your thoughts about the event.**

   Thoughts reflect the meaning or interpretation you have about what happened. It's very common to have difficulty in figuring out what your thoughts are about events that happen. So here are some questions to help you figure out what you think about what has occurred. Ask yourself these questions:

   - What just passed through my mind when the event happened?
   - What does this happening say about me as a person?
   - How will this event affect my future?
   - What's the worst thing about this event?
   - How will this event affect my life today?
   - How am I interpreting or what meaning am I making out of this event?

Table A-3	SAD Thought Tracker	
Feelings and Sensations	*Events*	*Thoughts or Interpretations*

SAD Thought Tracker and Reality Unscrambler Form

In this form, the SAD Thought Tracker combines with the Reality Unscrambler. Use it to make your thoughts more realistic and less distorted. See Chapter 10 for more information and an example of this technique. Here's how each section works:

✔ **Feelings and Sensations:** In the first column, write down both your body's sensations and a feeling word that describes those sensations. Also rate the feeling words for intensity from 1 (very mild) to 100 (extremely intense or severe).

✔ **Events:** In the second column, write down what you think may have triggered the feelings and sensations. Ask yourself what was going on.

✔ **Thoughts or Interpretations:** In the last column, record your thoughts about the event. Thoughts reflect the meaning or interpretation you have about what happened.

✔ **Initial Thoughts:** Briefly rewrite your initial thoughts from the thought tracker in the first column.

✔ **Reality Scramblers:** Refer to the Reality Scrambler list in Chapter 10 and jot down any reality scramblers that you think are contained within your thoughts.

✔ **Unscrambled Thoughts:** Write down thoughts that express a more realistic, less scrambled perspective on your initial thoughts.

✔ **Rating the Results:** In other words, take another look at your feelings and indicate whether they've changed. Express what you feel you got out of the exercise.

Table A-4	SAD Thought Tracker and Reality Unscrambler Form	
Feelings and Sensations	*Events*	*Thoughts or Interpretations*
Initial Thoughts	*Reality Scramblers*	*Unscrambled Thoughts*
Rating the Results:		

Activity Log

Keeping an activity log is one of the best first steps you can take if you have severe depression and you neglect important responsibilities or chores. The technique is straightforward and fairly simple. Follow these steps to fill out your activity log:

1. **Schedule one neglected activity for each day and write it in the second column of the form.**

   Make it a small activity at first.

2. **After you complete the activity, write down how it went and how you feel about accomplishing it in the last column of the form.**

See Chapter 14 for more information.

Table A-5	Activity Log	
Day	*Activity*	*Outcome*
M		
T		
W		
Th		
F		
Sa		
Su		

Critical State of Mind and Observing State of Mind Forms

In Chapter 18, we discuss how the mind has two very different states: One is evaluative, judgmental, and critical, while the other is observant and non-judgmental. Which one do you think feels better? We suggest the later. When you find yourself overly critical, try using this form to snap you out of it:

1. **Think about something that you've been evaluating negatively.**

2. **Write down each and every critical thought in the form under *Critical Thoughts.***

3. **Notice how you feel when you're finished and write those feelings down under *Feelings after Writing Critical Thoughts.***

4. **Think about what you just wrote.**

5. **Now connect with your senses and describe the same information from Steps 2 and 3 as objectively as you can.**

   Write these experiences as they come to you under *Observations, Sensations, and Experiences.* Don't worry about sentence structure, punctuation, or grammar.

6. **Notice how you feel now and jot these feelings down under *Feelings after Writing Observations and Experiences.***

Table A-6	Critical State of Mind
Critical Thoughts	
Feelings after Writing Critical Thoughts	

Table A-7	Observing State of Mind

Observations, Sensations, and Experiences

Feelings after Writing Observations and Experiences

Appendix B

SAD Resources for You

● ●

*I*n this appendix, we highlight some other seasonal affective disorder (SAD) sources for you. Although *Seasonal Affective Disorder For Dummies* is comprehensive and complete, sometimes reading other material is helpful, too. This list isn't intended to be exhaustive, and we're pretty sure that we may have missed a source or two, but nevertheless, we offer a variety of resources for your consideration.

Self-Help Books

✔ *Anxiety & Depression Workbook For Dummies* by Charles H. Elliott, PhD, and Laura L. Smith, PhD (Wiley)

✔ *Changing For Good: The Revolutionary Program that Explains the Six Stages of Change and Teaches You How to Free Yourself From Bad Habits* by James O. Prochaska, John C. Norcross, and Carlo C. DiClemente (William Morrow & Co., Inc.)

✔ *Depression For Dummies* by Laura L. Smith, PhD, and Charles H. Elliott, PhD (Wiley)

✔ *Feeling Better, Getting Better, Staying Better: Profound Self-Help Therapy for Your Emotions* by Albert Ellis (Impact Publishers)

✔ *Full Catastrophe Living: Using the Wisdom of Your Body and Mind to Face Stress, Pain, and Illness* by Jon Kabat-Zinn (Delta)

✔ *Mind Over Mood: Change How You Feel by Changing The Way You Think* by Dennis Greenberger and Christine A. Padesky (Guildford Press)

✔ *Overcoming Anxiety For Dummies* by Charles H. Elliott, PhD, and Laura L. Smith, PhD (Wiley)

✔ *Positive Options for Seasonal Affective Disorder (SAD): Self-Help and Treatment* by Fiona Marshall and Peter Cheevers (Hunter House Publishers)

✔ *The Feeling Good Handbook* by David D. Burns, MD (Plume)

✔ *Why Can't I Get What I Want? How to Stop Making the Same Old Mistakes and Start Living a Life You Can Love* by Charles H. Elliott, PhD, and Maureen Kirby Lassen (Davies-Black)

✔ *Winter Blues: Everything You Need to Know to Beat Seasonal Affective Disorder* by Norman E. Rosenthal (Guilford Press)

Web Sites

The Internet contains a vast array of information and resources about almost anything you can imagine. Unfortunately, some of the sources are unreliable. The following list represents organizations' Web sites we deem trustworthy. Check them out:

✔ **www.healthyminds.org:** The American Psychiatric Association provides information about SAD and other mental disorders at this site.

✔ **www.apa.org/pubinfo:** The American Psychological Association provides information about the treatment of, as well as interesting facts about, SAD and other emotional disorders.

✔ **www.nami.org:** The National Alliance for the Mentally Ill is a wonderful organization that serves as an advocate for people and families affected by SAD and other mental disorders. Information is available about the causes, prevalence, and treatments of mental disorders that affect children and adults.

✔ **www.nccam.nih.gov:** This site is run by the National Center for Complementary and Alternative Medicine. It's a government-sponsored site designed to provide information about alternative treatments for depression and other disorders. Most of the advice on this site is based on research (unlike other sites that focus on selling alternative medicine products).

✔ **www.nimh.nih.gov:** The National Institute of Mental Health reports on research about a wide variety of mental health issues. It also has an array of educational materials on SAD and depression and provides resources for researchers and practitioners in the field.

✔ **www.sada.org.uk:** The Seasonal Affective Disorder Association is an organization in Great Britain that provides information and support to people with SAD.

✔ **www.sltbr.org:** The Society for Light Treatment and Biological Rhythms is an international organization that encourages research in the area of light therapy and biological rhythms. Its Web site contains extensive information about SAD, light therapy, melatonin, and circadian rhythm disorders.

✔ **www.webmd.com:** WebMD provides a vast array of information about both physical and mental health issues (including SAD) and contains information about psychological treatments, drug therapy, and prevention.

Index

Notes

Notes

Notes

SINESS, CAREERS & PERSONAL FINANCE

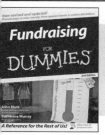

0-7645-9847-3

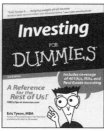

0-7645-2431-3

Also available:
- Business Plans Kit For Dummies
  0-7645-9794-9
- Economics For Dummies
  0-7645-5726-2
- Grant Writing For Dummies
  0-7645-8416-2
- Home Buying For Dummies
  0-7645-5331-3
- Managing For Dummies
  0-7645-1771-6
- Marketing For Dummies
  0-7645-5600-2

- Personal Finance For Dummies
  0-7645-2590-5*
- Resumes For Dummies
  0-7645-5471-9
- Selling For Dummies
  0-7645-5363-1
- Six Sigma For Dummies
  0-7645-6798-5
- Small Business Kit For Dummies
  0-7645-5984-2
- Starting an eBay Business For Dummies
  0-7645-6924-4
- Your Dream Career For Dummies
  0-7645-9795-7

OME & BUSINESS COMPUTER BASICS

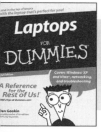

0-470-05432-8

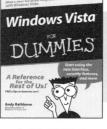

0-471-75421-8

Also available:
- Cleaning Windows Vista For Dummies
  0-471-78293-9
- Excel 2007 For Dummies
  0-470-03737-7
- Mac OS X Tiger For Dummies
  0-7645-7675-5
- MacBook For Dummies
  0-470-04859-X
- Macs For Dummies
  0-470-04849-2
- Office 2007 For Dummies
  0-470-00923-3

- Outlook 2007 For Dummies
  0-470-03830-6
- PCs For Dummies
  0-7645-8958-X
- Salesforce.com For Dummies
  0-470-04893-X
- Upgrading & Fixing Laptops For Dummies
  0-7645-8959-8
- Word 2007 For Dummies
  0-470-03658-3
- Quicken 2007 For Dummies
  0-470-04600-7

OD, HOME, GARDEN, HOBBIES, MUSIC & PETS

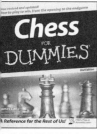

0-7645-8404-9

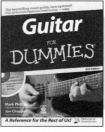

0-7645-9904-6

Also available:
- Candy Making For Dummies
  0-7645-9734-5
- Card Games For Dummies
  0-7645-9910-0
- Crocheting For Dummies
  0-7645-4151-X
- Dog Training For Dummies
  0-7645-8418-9
- Healthy Carb Cookbook For Dummies
  0-7645-8476-6
- Home Maintenance For Dummies
  0-7645-5215-5

- Horses For Dummies
  0-7645-9797-3
- Jewelry Making & Beading For Dummies
  0-7645-2571-9
- Orchids For Dummies
  0-7645-6759-4
- Puppies For Dummies
  0-7645-5255-4
- Rock Guitar For Dummies
  0-7645-5356-9
- Sewing For Dummies
  0-7645-6847-7
- Singing For Dummies
  0-7645-2475-5

TERNET & DIGITAL MEDIA

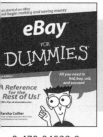

0-470-04529-9

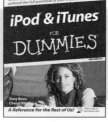

0-470-04894-8

Also available:
- Blogging For Dummies
  0-471-77084-1
- Digital Photography For Dummies
  0-7645-9802-3
- Digital Photography All-in-One Desk Reference For Dummies
  0-470-03743-1
- Digital SLR Cameras and Photography For Dummies
  0-7645-9803-1
- eBay Business All-in-One Desk Reference For Dummies
  0-7645-8438-3
- HDTV For Dummies
  0-470-09673-X

- Home Entertainment PCs For Dummies
  0-470-05523-5
- MySpace For Dummies
  0-470-09529-6
- Search Engine Optimization For Dummies
  0-471-97998-8
- Skype For Dummies
  0-470-04891-3
- The Internet For Dummies
  0-7645-8996-2
- Wiring Your Digital Home For Dummies
  0-471-91830-X

parate Canadian edition also available
parate U.K. edition also available

able wherever books are sold. For more information or to order direct: U.S. customers visit www.dummies.com or call 1-877-762-2974.
customers visit www.wileyeurope.com or call 0800 243407. Canadian customers visit www.wiley.ca or call 1-800-567-4797.

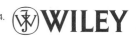

SPORTS, FITNESS, PARENTING, RELIGION & SPIRITUALITY

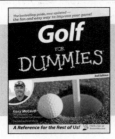

0-471-76871-5

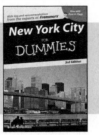

0-7645-7841-3

Also available:

✔ Catholicism For Dummies
0-7645-5391-7

✔ Exercise Balls For Dummies
0-7645-5623-1

✔ Fitness For Dummies
0-7645-7851-0

✔ Football For Dummies
0-7645-3936-1

✔ Judaism For Dummies
0-7645-5299-6

✔ Potty Training For Dummies
0-7645-5417-4

✔ Buddhism For Dummies
0-7645-5359-3

✔ Pregnancy For Dummies
0-7645-4483-7 †

✔ Ten Minute Tone-Ups For Dummies
0-7645-7207-5

✔ NASCAR For Dummies
0-7645-7681-X

✔ Religion For Dummies
0-7645-5264-3

✔ Soccer For Dummies
0-7645-5229-5

✔ Women in the Bible For Dummies
0-7645-8475-8

TRAVEL

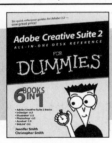

0-7645-7749-2

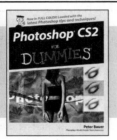

0-7645-6945-7

Also available:

✔ Alaska For Dummies
0-7645-7746-8

✔ Cruise Vacations For Dummies
0-7645-6941-4

✔ England For Dummies
0-7645-4276-1

✔ Europe For Dummies
0-7645-7529-5

✔ Germany For Dummies
0-7645-7823-5

✔ Hawaii For Dummies
0-7645-7402-7

✔ Italy For Dummies
0-7645-7386-1

✔ Las Vegas For Dummies
0-7645-7382-9

✔ London For Dummies
0-7645-4277-X

✔ Paris For Dummies
0-7645-7630-5

✔ RV Vacations For Dummies
0-7645-4442-X

✔ Walt Disney World & Orlando
For Dummies
0-7645-9660-8

GRAPHICS, DESIGN & WEB DEVELOPMENT

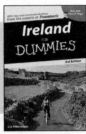

0-7645-8815-X

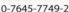

0-7645-9571-7

Also available:

✔ 3D Game Animation For Dummies
0-7645-8789-7

✔ AutoCAD 2006 For Dummies
0-7645-8925-3

✔ Building a Web Site For Dummies
0-7645-7144-3

✔ Creating Web Pages For Dummies
0-470-08030-2

✔ Creating Web Pages All-in-One Desk
Reference For Dummies
0-7645-4345-8

✔ Dreamweaver 8 For Dummies
0-7645-9649-7

✔ InDesign CS2 For Dummies
0-7645-9572-5

✔ Macromedia Flash 8 For Dummies
0-7645-9691-8

✔ Photoshop CS2 and Digital
Photography For Dummies
0-7645-9580-6

✔ Photoshop Elements 4 For Dummies
0-471-77483-9

✔ Syndicating Web Sites with RSS Feeds
For Dummies
0-7645-8848-6

✔ Yahoo! SiteBuilder For Dummies
0-7645-9800-7

NETWORKING, SECURITY, PROGRAMMING & DATABASES

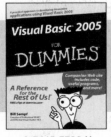

0-7645-7728-X

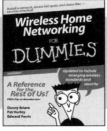

0-471-74940-0

Also available:

✔ Access 2007 For Dummies
0-470-04612-0

✔ ASP.NET 2 For Dummies
0-7645-7907-X

✔ C# 2005 For Dummies
0-7645-9704-3

✔ Hacking For Dummies
0-470-05235-X

✔ Hacking Wireless Networks
For Dummies
0-7645-9730-2

✔ Java For Dummies
0-470-08716-1

✔ Microsoft SQL Server 2005 For Dummies
0-7645-7755-7

✔ Networking All-in-One Desk Reference
For Dummies
0-7645-9939-9

✔ Preventing Identity Theft For Dummies
0-7645-7336-5

✔ Telecom For Dummies
0-471-77085-X

✔ Visual Studio 2005 All-in-One Desk
Reference For Dummies
0-7645-9775-2

✔ XML For Dummies
0-7645-8845-1

ALTH & SELF-HELP

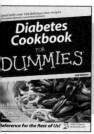

0-7645-8450-2

0-7645-4149-8

Also available:

- Bipolar Disorder For Dummies
  0-7645-8451-0
- Chemotherapy and Radiation For Dummies
  0-7645-7832-4
- Controlling Cholesterol For Dummies
  0-7645-5440-9
- Diabetes For Dummies
  0-7645-6820-5* †
- Divorce For Dummies
  0-7645-8417-0 †

- Fibromyalgia For Dummies
  0-7645-5441-7
- Low-Calorie Dieting For Dummies
  0-7645-9905-4
- Meditation For Dummies
  0-471-77774-9
- Osteoporosis For Dummies
  0-7645-7621-6
- Overcoming Anxiety For Dummies
  0-7645-5447-6
- Reiki For Dummies
  0-7645-9907-0
- Stress Management For Dummies
  0-7645-5144-2

JCATION, HISTORY, REFERENCE & TEST PREPARATION

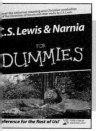

0-7645-8381-6

0-7645-9554-7

Also available:

- The ACT For Dummies
  0-7645-9652-7
- Algebra For Dummies
  0-7645-5325-9
- Algebra Workbook For Dummies
  0-7645-8467-7
- Astronomy For Dummies
  0-7645-8465-0
- Calculus For Dummies
  0-7645-2498-4
- Chemistry For Dummies
  0-7645-5430-1
- Forensics For Dummies
  0-7645-5580-4

- Freemasons For Dummies
  0-7645-9796-5
- French For Dummies
  0-7645-5193-0
- Geometry For Dummies
  0-7645-5324-0
- Organic Chemistry I For Dummies
  0-7645-6902-3
- The SAT I For Dummies
  0-7645-7193-1
- Spanish For Dummies
  0-7645-5194-9
- Statistics For Dummies
  0-7645-5423-9

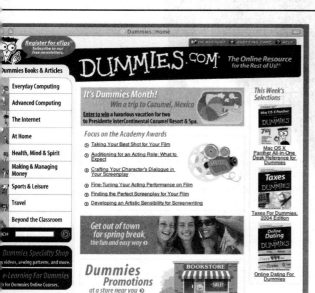

Get smart @ dummies.com®

- **Find a full list of Dummies titles**
- **Look into loads of FREE on-site articles**
- **Sign up for FREE eTips e-mailed to you weekly**
- **See what other products carry the Dummies name**
- **Shop directly from the Dummies bookstore**
- **Enter to win new prizes every month!**

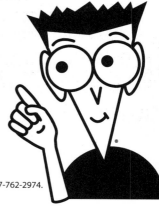

arate Canadian edition also available

arate U.K. edition also available

ble wherever books are sold. For more information or to order direct: U.S. customers visit www.dummies.com or call 1-877-762-2974.
ustomers visit www.wileyeurope.com or call 0800 243407. Canadian customers visit www.wiley.ca or call 1-800-567-4797.

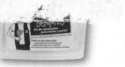
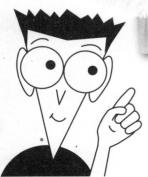